Language Therapy Space:
Teaching English as a Foreign Language to the Visually Impaired

POLISH STUDIES IN ENGLISH LANGUAGE AND LITERATURE

Edited by Jacek Fisiak

VOL. 38

PETER LANG
EDITION

Beata Wyszyńska

Language Therapy Space: Teaching English as a Foreign Language to the Visually Impaired

PETER LANG EDITION

Bibliographic Information published by the Deutsche Nationalbibliothek
The Deutsche Nationalbibliothek lists this publication in the Deutsche Nationalbibliografie; detailed bibliographic data is available in the internet at http://dnb.d-nb.de.

This Publication was financially supported by the University of Social Sciences.

UNIVERSITY OF SOCIAL SCIENCES

ISSN 1436-7513
ISBN 978-3-631-66845-0 (Print)
E-ISBN 978-3-653-06077-5 (E-PDF)
E-ISBN 978-3-631-69499-2 (EPUB)
E-ISBN 978-3-631-69500-5 (MOBI)
DOI 10.3726/978-3-653-06077-5

Peter Lang – Frankfurt am Main · Bern · Bruxelles · New York · Oxford · Warszawa · Wien

This publication has been peer reviewed.

www.peterlang.com

To my beloved Parents

Acknowledgements

I wish to thank Professor Jerzy Zybert for helping me attain clarity of mind and belief in my inner flow.

I would like to thank my students for teaching me that sight is a gift.

I am grateful to Bartosz Zdziech for psychological support.

Table of Contents

List of figures

List of tables

List of appendices

Abbreviations and typographic conventions

ACB – American Council of the Blind
AER – Association for Education and Rehabilitation of the Blind and Visually Impaired
AFB – American Foundation for the Blind
BES – Behavioural Engagement System
BIS – Behavioural Inhibition System
BSM – Brain Linkage Method
CBT – Cognitive-Behavioural Therapy
EABCT – European Association for Behavioural and Cognitive Therapies
ICEVI – International Council for Education of People with Visual Impairment
LAD – Language Acquisition Device
NA – Negative Affect
NLP – No Light Perception
PA – Positive Affect
PANAS – Positive and Negative Affect Schedule
PLT – Psycho-Linguistic Therapy "Touching the World"
RNIB – Royal National Institute for the Blind
TPR – Total Physical Response
TSR – Tactile Structure Repetition

Introduction

Teaching a language to visually impaired people involves complex challenges which may be effectively met by combining and synthesising knowledge from a broad range of fields.

Above all, blind students need to feel that the axis of their world is stable and reliable, and to accept it. The blind need the spur of a dynamic force that will elicit an active language response from them. Indeed, they need it more than other learners do because, for some of them at any rate, placidity is a millstone which anchors them comfortably in the backwaters of life, whereas what they need is to be encouraged to sail forth into life's main current (Burklen, 1985).

As a teacher of English, I have been particularly attracted to matters concerning visual impairments in relation to teaching English as a foreign language. Such inspiration helped me create the method addressed to the visually handicapped – the Re-charged Direct Method within the psycho-linguistic therapy "Touching the World". Following John Dewey's theory (2007), that any educational process has two aspects – one psychological and one sociological – and that of these two, the psychological is deeper, I could not imagine teaching English without the psychological context. In my view, without insight into the psychological structure and activities of the individual, the educative process will be haphazard and arbitrary.

When I started to observe and inquire into visually impaired students I felt a real need to understand the difficulties of visual impairments, and accept them as normal standards, thinking that the achievement of normal standards is miraculous. Initially, my plan was to teach English in the most effective and creative way. In doing so I found myself alone in the jungle of my students' problems, their blindness, and their low level (or outright absence) of English. Confusion and uncertainty were excellent beginning points for the process of discovery. I found teaching the visually impaired to be a complex and difficult philosophy. Questions of existence and the need for exploring them were considered on diverse levels of the therapy process, where they involved combinations of philosophical, psychological, ethical, and behavioural perspectives.

Following these observations and inspired by relevant authors I set out to develop a PhD study: ***Language Therapy Space: Teaching English as a foreign language to the visually impaired.***

The psycho-linguistic therapy (PLT) "Touching the World" is first and foremost a process of teaching English as a foreign language directed to visually impaired adult students; a kind of two-path case study that joins linguistic and mental layers.

The language basis was focused on the Direct Method issues that were transformed into the Re-charged Direct Method, and enriched with diverse types of supports: sand and water experiments based on tactile perception. The mental layer aimed at involving the whole person within the process of positive and negative affect change, in consideration of physically and mentally conditioned factors, taught on several different levels within the edu-kinaesthetic area and the Brain Linkage Method.

This dissertation consists of two parts, theoretical and empirical, and seven chapters. The sequence of chapters is not accidental; the chain of their appearance is purposeful – each chapter constitutes a base for the next. The first part of this thesis is devoted to theoretical considerations of tyflology, axilogy, psychology and their connections with linguistics. It thus prepares the ground for discussing the empirical research. The theoretical part covers four chapters (Chapters 1–4) which emphasise the background of designing the psycho-linguistic therapy "Touching the World", rooted in the Re-charged Direct Method, based on visual disorder classification, the psychology of blindness, theory of language learning, perspectives on personality, and the notions of motivation and flow. The second part of the study, the empirical part, is made up of three chapters (Chapters 5–7). They present and discuss practical implications of the Re-charged Direct Method within the PLT experiment, and contain research methodology, data collection, recommendations, and implications for further research into pedagogy for the visually impaired, with analysis of the implementations of two-layered-triangulation.

Chapter **one** discusses the issues related to visual disorder classifications, involving the field of sensory compensation employed in the impairment. I found considerations of the kinaesthetic deficit correlated with the concepts of behavioural-environmental codependence, salient to be mentioned. Teaching English to the visually handicapped is analysed within the cohesion of receptive and productive skills and special didactic devices.

Chapter **two**, then, comprises diverse mental therapy areas, focused on the intensity of positive and negative emotions, implemented in the PLT correlation with various psychodynamic therapies, sand and water clues, leading to the development of motivation – in its intrinsic and extrinsic layers – providing the achievement of the self-acceptance model of being, mentioning differentiated perspectives on personality issues, through the rule of three-layer intelligence structure. Measuring the intensity of affects through the Positive and Negative Affect Schedule (PANAS questionnaire) is involved in group therapy issues. Theoretical distinguishing between emotion, feeling, and affect is also emphasised.

Chapter **three** presents the linguistic field of the therapy, based on theories of language learning, Direct Method issues, the Audiolingual Method, and Total Physical Response. The notions of approach, method, and technique are considered to be crucial in relation to foreign language teaching and learning. The chapter analyses language as a means of expressing emotions, rooted in its social and psychological contexts.

Chapter **four** is devoted to exploring the Re-charged Direct Method and its place in the PLT structure. The mutual relationship between grammar-water and lexis-sand experiments is demonstrated on the basis of the implementation of the Re-charged Direct Method, with supportive issues of the tactile repetition structures represented by "the ping-pong sentence structure", "the tactile knots technique", and "vocabulary movement" – focusing on the word segmentation process. Of secondary importance is the sandtray therapy that corresponds to the Brain Linkage Method, edu-kinaesthetic brain gym or "controlled breathing" practice.

Chapter **five** discusses practical implications of the Re-charged Direct Method rooted in "Touching the World". The involvement of haptic techniques correlates with classroom design, emphasising creative and efficient aspects of the foreign language teaching-learning process to the visually impaired in the PLT.

In chapter **six** special attention is paid to the research conducted among visually impaired students. The research methodology is considered through case study principles via the methodology instrumentation (a PANAS questionnaire, placement and achievement tests in L2) and the analysis of data collection. This chapter commences with an elaboration of the hypotheses employed in the study and the involvement of dependent variables: achievements in L2, the intensity of positive and negative affects and the independent variable: visual impairment. The discussion of the research results is concluded with the claim that building a bridge between mental and linguistic areas leads to emotional balance, the intensity of positive effects, and the language communicative approach in parallel.

This thesis closes with conclusions and a discussion of findings having implications for further research into pedagogy for the visually handicapped in chapter **seven.** Possible directions for future research are also indicated.

Samples of training materials, testing tools and supplementary measures are provided in the **appendices.** Thus, they contain relevant and hopefully noteworthy additions which had been included in the main body of the dissertation.

This dissertation reflects my interest in issues pertaining to developing successful communicative linguistic competences within psychologically-based therapy, leading to the achievement of emotionally conditioned balance, an increase in positive activation and a decrease in negative, through the therapeutic acquisition of a second language.

It is my hope that the analysis included in this thesis will provide an added value to the current methodological issues directed toward visually impaired students.

May the theoretical and empirical matters raised in this dissertation prove enlightening.

Part One: Theoretical Backdrops and Considerations

Chapter One: Visual impairments – physical, psychological and didactic consequences

1.0. Introductory remarks

This chapter presents and explains some of the main terms and concepts that are employed throughout this thesis. In chapter one special attention is paid to visual impairment that entails the loss of physical, emotional, and mental control, as this is regarded as one of the most distressing by-products of the crisis and conflict of "self". The consequences of the disability are seen through the expressions of pejorative emotions – psychological blockers – which students undergo.

The chapter presents classifications of visual impairments with special attention given to the sensory compensation aspect, correlated with the kinaesthetic deficit. I herein clearly indicate the physical obstacles to communicative approach achievements that accompany the teaching-learning process directed to visually impaired students. I have found the issue of special didactic devices to be crucial in this dissertation.

1.1. Visual disorder classification

The extent of visual disability depends upon the physical sensory impairment of the student's eyes, the age of the student at the onset of visual impairment, and the way in which that impairment occurred.

Visual impairment is usually described within three parameters: visual acuity, field of vision and functional efficiency (Krzeszowski, 2012):

- *Visual acuity* is measured by reading letters of different sizes, or by detecting the orientation of gratings of progressively narrower spacing. The results of such tests are expressed in terms of the distance at which the individual can read a letter compared with the norm for that size of letter. Thus 6/60 means that a person can see letters at 6 metres which can normally be distinguished at 60 metres.
- *Visual field* is the area that can be seen without moving one's eyes when looking straight ahead: a visual field of about 160 to 180 degrees is considered typical. A restricted visual field means the inability to see peripherally: it is often referred to as tunnel vision. The simplest method of testing is to bring

a snapping finger from one side of the ear to the front, move it up and down, and mark the position where the person can see the finger.

- *Functional efficiency* refers to the vision available to a person for the performance of everyday tasks according to his/her needs, motivation or expectations.

Students who have the same visual condition may use their sight quite differently. There is no "typical" vision impaired student (Pelczarska, 1997). Some students may have vision problems other than or in addition to reduced visual acuity or restricted visual field, including blind spots in their visual fields, high or low sensitivity to normal levels of light, difficulty distinguishing colours or contrast, or a combination of several of these conditions. The type of visual impairment that a student has is also a major factor in his or her visual functioning. With some eye disorders, vision may actually fluctuate from day to day or throughout the day during different lighting and environmental conditions. Even stable vision conditions may be temporarily influenced by such factors as lighting, fatigue, attention, and emotions. In addition, many students have additional disabilities that accompany their visual impairments, such as cognitive impairments or learning disabilities.

In working with visually impaired students one encounters a variety of related terms (Sękowska, 1981). Individuals who are not totally blind but have visual impairments that cannot be corrected to normal with regular eyeglasses or contact lenses are referred to as having low vision. The term legal blindness is related to the visual ability of individuals who have visual acuity of 6/60 or worse in the better corrected eye, or who have visual field restricted to 20 degrees or less at the widest point. Many students who are legally blind have a significant amount of usable vision and can often read regular or large print. Total blindness is the complete lack of form and light perception and is clinically recorded as NLP, an abbreviation for "no light perception". The majority of people who are blind have some useful sight even if it is only light perception: 4% are totally blind.

The following classification for students with visual impairment reflects educational purposes related to appropriate classroom accommodations (Spungin, 2008):

- low vision – students use their vision as the primary sensory channel,
- functionally blind – students use limited vision for functional tasks, but need their tactile and auditory channels for learning,
- totally blind – students use tactile and auditory channels for learning and functional tasks.

The next classification system is based on the advent of the visual impairment itself (Dycht, 2005):

- congenital – occurs during foetal development at birth or immediately following birth; visual impairment is present before visual memory has been established,
- adventitious – occurs after having normal vision either through a hereditary condition or trauma; visual memory may remain.

Students with congenital visual impairment typically have more difficulty mastering visually strengthened concepts such as spacious orientation and many environmental concepts.

It is essential to know that visually impaired students differ in their ability to use their vision. Two students may have the same visual acuity, visual fields, and other clinical measurements, but one may use sight to perform the same tasks that the other does more efficiently using his or her other senses. These individual differences affect the way the student obtains information and learns.

Visual impairment is often correlated with hearing disorder (Rezenand and Hausman, 1985). Two terms are used to refer to hearing impairments: deaf and hard-of-hearing. Deaf means a hearing loss that prevents a person from understanding speech. People who are deaf have little functional hearing even with a hearing aid; they do not use hearing as their primary sense of gaining information. Hard-of-hearing means that a person can process information from sounds and often can benefit from the amplification provided by hearing aids.

1.2. Sensory compensation

Blind students are visually impaired but their other senses are intact. The absence of sight heightens other areas of sensory perception. This is referred to as sensory compensation, which is the ability of intact senses to compensate for the lack of one or more of them. Do the auditory skills of the visually impaired compensate for their loss of sight? Blind people have a highly developed sense of hearing. As the thinking goes, the five senses work in concert with one another, such that the loss of one is compensated by increased sensitivity in the remaining four (Gougoux et al., 2009).

The issue of sensory compensation may be elaborated within two perception areas: hearing and touch. Hearing appears before touch is recognised. A blind person can become quite adept at using echolocation – identifying an object by the sound or echo it makes – while moving through the world around him/her. According to the RNIB, the use of reflected sound helps the blind explore and manipulate aspects of the sound world. Visually impaired individuals may make clicking noises to note the changes in sound as the distance between them and obstacles shifts (Sękowska, 1981). The largest area of the brain's surface is devoted to the hand or the skin, which the blind use to access information. For instance, many blind individuals feel changes in temperature as they near a window or wall and thus rely on their enhanced senses of touch to recognise the environment (Bandler, 1985). Sensory compensation employs the involvement of the haptic analyser, and this may be considered on two diverse levels: a person feels his/her touch and feels being touched. Touch itself incorporates mental features of tactile feeling that leads to haptic mental rotation. Touch ought to be analysed as a passive or active experience. Passive touch is limited to an impression of touch that results in the feeling of warmth or cold. Active touch is compared with movement (Burklen, 1985).

Until recently there had been little empirical evidence that blind people really do benefit from sensory compensation. At the Montreal Neurological Institute at Canada's McGill University, Robert Zatorre, a neuroscientist and experimental psychologist, put popular perceptions to the test. Their results confirmed expectations and also yielded some exciting surprises (Gougoux et al., 2009).

The study began simply enough, with groups of blind and sighted subjects alike tested on pitch perception (how high or low a note is) and position perception (where in space a sound is located). In line with expectations, blind subjects scored better than their sighted counterparts. However, an unforeseen observation arose: the people who had been blind since birth were the ones who scored best. In fact, the scores correlated directly to the point in life at which each subject had lost his or her eyesight. Those born blind had the best performance, followed by subjects who became blind at the age of four or five. Among those blinded at ten or later, there was little to no difference at all compared to the sighted group. "What this tells us is that there is plasticity in the brain", says Zatorre. "That is, when we are young we can actually change around the way neurons work, and reorganize brain function to suit our survival needs. But as we get older, the brain becomes more or less fixed in terms of sensory perception" (Gougoux et al., 2009:2967). In the second test, subjects had one ear plugged and were then asked to locate where sounds were coming from in a room with hidden speakers. Knowing that the brain compares input from both ears to locate sounds, the researcher did not expect anyone to score highly – yet half of the blind people evinced impressive accuracy.

These results are probably the best evidence of one sense being compensated by another. Zatorre believes that the blind people who scored well were gleaning highly specific location information from the sound as it was bouncing off their outer ears. While the cartilage in everyone's outer ear has a unique topography of folds, these subjects were using the ear's features to a far greater effect. The sound was there for all to hear, but these subjects had become extremely sensitive to the information it provided.

Another surprise came when the researcher used positron emission tomography (PET scan), which indicates brain activity during the performance of various tasks. Zatorre knew that every subject would show activity in the auditory cortex, since that is where the brain processes sound. But for some subjects, the PET revealed activity in the visual cortex, where the brain processes sight. The people with visual activity were the same ones who had shown that particular ability to locate sound with one ear blocked. "We learned that the part of the brain that normally handles vision does not just die or atrophy without input", confirms Zatorre, "it somehow adds functionality to process subtle auditory information" (Gougoux et al., 2009:2969).

These startling PET-scan results are a testament to the incredible adaptive abilities of the brain. It can practically be rewired in our earliest years, and areas of the brain previously understood to have discrete functions can sometimes be recruited to help accommodate a loss.

The portions of the brain at birth that deal with vision, hearing and all other senses are connected, according to Belin (2000). As a sighted child grows, these connections begin to separate from one another until independent centres in the brain control each of the senses. Belin says these connections might remain in a blind infant, and the job of processing sound might be shared by both the visual cortex and auditory processing centres. If a person loses his/her sight during childhood or adulthood, the connections might have already separated because myelin, the fatty sheath surrounding affected nerves, develops rapidly in youth. Using neuroimaging tools, researchers have found that while regions in the brain that deal with vision are smaller in blind individuals than in those of the sighted, other nonvisual areas are larger. Blindness causes structural changes in the brain, indicating that the brain may reorganize itself functionally in order to adapt to a loss in sensory input. Areas in the brain responsible for memory, hearing and the remaining senses are all enlarged. (Czerwińska, 2007).

To conclude, a blind life is different from a sighted life, it is not lesser, reinforcing the idea that other senses are not only affected but enhanced by blindness.

1.3. Psychological and physical consequences of the disorder

The blind are ordinary people who find themselves in extraordinarily unfortunate circumstances. Ordinary behaviour, in the sense of the behaviour of the majority of an unselected sample of people in extraordinary circumstances, may not necessarily be the same as behaviour in ordinary circumstances. In this respect, it would seem that what would generally be regarded as extraordinary behaviour is just ordinary behaviour in the peculiar circumstances of blindness, and so the concept of two different standards of normality, one for the sighted majority and other for the blind minority, appears worthy of mention.

Blindness is among the most severe of all forms of disabilities. Without vision, people are cut off from a major segment of the social and physical environment to which they must adapt. This creates problems for mobility and everyday skilled activities for which vision is important. At the same time, in relating to other people, the blind can only guess the meanings and intentions of non-verbal communication, along with the social context in which these occur. Blindness may therefore create formidable social and psychological problems for the individual. These problems are compounded by the fear that this handicap produces in others and the unreasonable attitudes and reactions of sighted people to blindness (Sękowska, 1981).

For people who are born blind, living without sight is a normal part of their lives. But for people who have to learn to cope with going blind later in life, it appears to be a huge adjustment. Acquired blindness seems to be potentially more emotionally disturbing than the congenital forms of the impairment (Cooper, 1976). This may be because those with the acquired handicap are fully aware of what they are missing. They also bring to the handicap the prejudices that they had before losing their vision.

Social skills

Communication is the primary area in which students with visual impairments experience difficulty (Norris, 1972). Overcoming a student's visual limitation requires unique and individual techniques based on that student's particular visual impairment and his/her communication skills.

Low vision and blindness may have an influence on social skills, effective understanding, and nonverbal or body language behaviour. In addition, dependence in all areas of development affects a student's behaviour and the behaviour of others towards the visually impaired. Social skills are important to a student's overall success. Students need instructions and feedback in appropriate ways of interacting with others, such as initiating a conversation without eye contact, age-appropriate ways of sitting and standing, and facial expressions. Students with visual impairments cannot see nonverbal forms of communication, so they miss out on the information and feelings displayed with a look, a nod, a smile, or a shrug.

The visually impaired focus on diverse abilities to develop the capacity to interact with other people, something that is an essential part of daily life and ranges from maintaining eye contact to greeting people with a handshake, as these social interchanges form the foundation of personal and business relationships. Daily living skills which the sighted learn through incidental observations may need to be taught to visually impaired students. For students with visual impairments, practical skills include not just performing tasks, but arranging for assistance when it seems appropriate.

Self-esteem

It is one of the aims of education to develop self-esteem or self-acceptance, something especially difficult to achieve for a person suffering from a handicap such as visual impairment, which makes him/her different from the majority and makes it difficult for him/her to participate fully in all activities and often puts him/her at a disadvantage vis-à-vis those to which he/she is admitted. In other words, his/her gregarious tendencies may easily be thwarted. And so it is that in an unplanned environment a blind person may easily grow up introverted, lethargic and abnormally docile. Students who are visually impaired are sensitive to teasing, criticism, or negative stereotyping from others. According to Greenberg (Burklen, 1985), the blind evince a high rate of neurotic factors such as a low level of self-realization, lack of faith, and a tendency to take their own opinions for granted.

There are two basic ways in which the visually impaired can deal with their problems: they can minimise its detrimental effects and demand to be treated on equal terms with the non-handicapped, or they can call for special treatment. Each strategy has an extreme version: denial that any problem exists, and resentment against such terms as impairment, or a desire for segregation from the general population, thus removing the need to compete, and so to risk failure (Gale, 1984).

Considering secondary consequences that derive not from blindness itself but from the way the visually impaired are treated by the sighted, it is therefore not surprising that behaviour of the kind that can reasonably be ascribed to an inferiority complex is fairly common among the blind. Career education is another critical area for the visually impaired. They are unemployed and underemployed. They often do not understand what jobs people do or how they complete them because they cannot observe them doing so. They need concrete, real-life experiences and information on a wide variety of jobs and the specific tasks required to perform them. They also need to be exposed from an early age and throughout their education to actual work sites and places of employment.

Codependence

Codependent tendencies are awakened by the physical and mental involvement in the impairment of the visually impaired, their relatives, and the environment around them. This kind of behavioural-environmental codependence appears in a triangulation of relationships. Families with a visually impaired member are physically and mentally affected by the consequences of the disability. Those who deal with handicapped people may be tempted to patronize or overprotect them (Gale, 1984). Unfortunately, such families may exhibit too much tension, an accompanying lack of meaningful communication and support, a discouraging atmosphere, and an inability for each member to develop and grow in a positive way.

I observed families of the blind that were involved in the activities of taking care of their blind adult children. Parents were caught in a kind of vicious circle, causing pain and destructive patterns in their relationships. They felt responsible for their visually impaired children's lives. They live their lives caring more for their children than for themselves, sometimes to the exclusion of "self being".

Kinaesthetic deficit

The next issue that corresponds with a physical consequence of the visual impairment is a kinaesthetic deficit. It should be noted that the environment of a blind person is much more restricted than that of a sighted one. Apart from sounds, which are in general difficult to identify without the aid of sight, his/her experience is limited to what he/she can touch and to kinaesthetic sensations resulting from his/her own muscular movements.

Low vision and blindness impact movement and the quality of motor skills. It has become increasingly apparent that totally and partially blind people possess deficiencies in their awareness of the environment. For some, it is such a problem that they never become familiar enough with the world in which they live, interact and learn. People with complete blindness or low vision have a difficult time self-navigating outside well-known environments. In fact, physical movement is one of the biggest challenges for the blind. Blind people must learn every detail about the home environment. Large obstacles must remain in one location to prevent injury. They may need to learn such spatial concepts as 'above', 'below' and 'next to' in relation to themselves and others and may need to develop a sense of how the individual parts of an object actually constitute a whole.

The visually impaired are forced to cooperate with a kinaesthetic deficit through the process of orientation and mobility development. Orientation refers to the ability to know where a person is located in the structure of the environment, while mobility refers to the ability to travel safely and independently, using various techniques or assistive devices, including becoming familiar with the environment, using a hand to trail along the walls of a room or hallway, using a white cane or other mobility devices, walking with a sighted guide, following a teacher or another student, using the other person's movements as visual cues.

Students develop a better understanding of their position in space through distinct environmental features, such as differences in the textures of floor coverings. Visual contrast in the environment can assist students who have low vision.

Blindisms

Some people with visual disorders also develop repetitive stereotypic movements commonly referred to as blindisms, such as rocking, eye poking, hand waving, making extra or rhythmic movements, drooping their heads, or making inappropriate sounds. Activities that provide and promote movement may discourage undesirable behaviour such as blindisms (Czerwińska, 2007).

Summing up, the visually impaired are taught to function through their basic body image and spatial concepts involving sensory awareness and a variety of travel skills gained in both indoor and outdoor environments.

1.4. Teaching the visually handicapped

Sensory impairments can have serious educational implications. Students who are blind and partly deaf have unique educational needs that can be accommodated with the assistance of material and environmental modifications and specific curriculum content. Often, the titanic obstacle to success is the negative attitudes of the sensory handicapped, their relatives, or just the environment around them. According to Jordan (Hainninen, 1990:58), an attitude that is making a difference today is that "the sensory impaired can do anything hearing or sighted people can do … except hear or see". His words speak broadly for a movement towards empowerment in which impaired people take control of their lives and demand active roles in the decision-making that affects them.

The impact of visual impairments on a teaching-learning process is very much a function of the severity of the condition (the degree of vision loss and its causes) and the age at which the student's vision was reduced. Modifications for students should be determined individually using assessment data: that is, they should not be based solely on vision status classification.

Students with visual impairments frequently may not have had as much access to information about their environment as some of the sighted. Their knowledge may be fragmented and incomplete because of their lack of visual information. As the sighted person moves through the learning process, he/she progresses through three levels of attainment: concrete, functional and abstract. This is the path the sighted person follows to form a conceptual framework. The blind person is at the concrete level of object perception. As he/she grows, his/her experiences and familiarity with objects increase, and he/she begins to relate to them on the functional level. However, the visually impaired usually have limited success in progressing to the abstract level. Because of the absence of vision and, therefore, reduced effectiveness of the tactual sense, the blind person seems to function primarily on the concrete and functional level. The blind are limited in what they can learn from this tactual manipulation of objects, in that the information they receive will not allow them to perceive the depth, intricacy or totality that are the essence of the object. Similarly, sounds – unless they are attached to meaningful and understood sources – will fade into meaninglessness or nothingness (Czerwińska, 2007).

The goals to which learning is directed are the same for the blind as for the sighted student, but differences occur in his/her manner of working with them. In the absence of sight the student has to depend very much upon other senses. Non-verbal communication goes compatibly with verbal, on the parallel levels of haptics (touch), olfactics (smell) and vocalics (voice). The degree of impairment and the student's background and training will affect the usefulness of the various strategies (Snyder and Kesselman, 1972).

During the psycho-linguistic therapy "Touching the World" I was forced to understand the visual conditions of the visually impaired. I was not aware of the medical implication of students' blindness and how much residual vision a person had. For this reason I found the following set of questions essential in my thesis. First and foremost, understanding the degrees of blindness and the background of the disability appeared crucial for designing a therapy (Burklen, 1985).

- Is the person totally blind?
- Does he/she have some sight left?
- What amount of residual vision does the blind person have?
- Should such residual vision be utilised to the maximum?
- How long has the student been blind?
- What is the background of the student's disorder?
- How and when did he/she become blind?
- Is he/she a Braille reader? (only a fraction of the blind are)

If the student became blind when he/she was eight or nine, he/she has a certain visual memory. A person will conceive ideas and images differently from someone who was blind at birth. Those who go blind in adult life also have difficulty in learning to read Braille.

For the purpose of promoting independence during the teaching-learning process, visually impaired students should be allowed to rely on themselves whenever possible. The student will also need to learn to ask for and accept assistance for certain tasks. In addition to the student being inculcated with a feeling of self-worth, he/she should be encouraged to offer assistance to other members of the group as well. It is essential to remember that safety practices must be balanced with the student's need to be independent.

An "independence programme" ought to be considered through various issues (Hainninen, 1990):

- encouraging the visually impaired student to move about the classroom to obtain materials or information seems to be crucial. The student will know his or her own needs, and his or her method of compensating will soon become a part of classroom routines. However, it is helpful for the student to be oriented to the classroom and for materials to be organised consistently in areas where the student can easily find them,
- keeping instructional materials in a consistent, specific place so the student knows where to find them easily,
- seating students with vision problems with their backs to windows or other sources of light to avoid glare on materials; reducing glare and visual distractions as much as possible,
- seating blind students with hearing impairment near the teacher, at the centre of arrangements, and arranging seating so that distracting noises are kept to a minimum for students with hearing problems,
- reducing unnecessary noise to help students focus on the content of instructional presentations,
- creating contrast with dark-lined paper and soft or felt-tip pens, helping students with vision problems to better discern information,
- speaking slowly and emphasising clear articulation rather than loudness when speaking,
- using complete sentences to provide additional context during conversations or instructional presentations,
- verbalising texts and describing pictures,
- narrating nonverbal actions or scenes,
- using auditory cues referring to objects in the classroom and during instructional presentations,

- being precise in giving directions or describing things,
- during group discussions, having one student speak at a time, and using the name of the speaker to facilitate communication and understanding,
- encouraging independent activities to teach social skills.

Meeting the didactic needs of students with low vision requires modifications to environmental and instructional materials as well as special equipment that will enhance a student's ability to acquire information. Environmental modifications such as additional lighting and special seating arrangements may be required (Majewski, 1983). The teacher of visually impaired students should be able to help identify the best seating arrangement for a particular student. If a student has a severely restricted visual field (tunnel vision), a seat farther back may be a better choice. Glare may cause discomfort or interfere with students' ability to read, some individuals with low vision prefer seats that face away from the window. Others prefer seats close to the window to get more natural light and avoid reflections off a shiny chalkboard or other surface. Considering demonstrations given during a lesson, visually handicapped students can be seated in a location that maximises his or her ability to see or follow what is being presented.

Moreover, material modifications such as adapting print material to promote maximum contrast, minimal visual distractions, and special size requirements may also be essential. The material should be prepared in alternate formats, such as in Braille, large-print, or an audio or electronic format. However, many visually impaired students can use books with regular-size type. They may need to bring books closer to their eyes, use optical devices, such as magnifiers, or alter the position of the reading material so they can see it better. They may also require more time to complete their assignments. It is usually considered acceptable for students with low vision to take time and a half and for those who read Braille to take twice the time.

Students with vision impairments rely on listening as a primary means of obtaining information. Focusing on a sound source and analysing oral information, listening skills are taught to help them cope with communication problems caused by vision disability.

The following tips correlate with developing writing skills (Spungin, 2008):

- Students with low vision may use bold-line paper, felt-tip pens, and other tools that increase the contrast and/or size of their writing to make it more visible.
- Students with low vision may benefit from using a reading stand to bring the paper closer to their eyes, rather than bending over a desk.
- Students with low vision write larger letters; they should write in a size that they are able to reread.

Students with low vision may read regular-print texts with or without the help of optical and non-optical devices or the use of large-print materials. In some cases, they may also use Braille.

The visually impaired need to develop certain essential skills. These skills are taught as part of a specialised and vital area of study known as the expanded core curriculum that consists of (Spungin, 2008):

- compensatory skills – including many basic skills that visually impaired students need to have access to information; they are the skills needed to participate fully in their general education subjects – the core curriculum – as well as general communication skills;
- functional academic skills – relating to the skills needed to accomplish daily living tasks, such as reading signs or paying bills;
- communication modes – refering to the methods, techniques of reading and writing that students use for literacy tasks, such as Braille reading and writing.

Blindness increases the difficulties usually encountered in any learning process. Therefore, the teacher of the blind must take particular care to ensure that the steps in any learning process are carefully graded. The student's readiness to tackle difficulties also depends on his/her attitude towards failure. Fear of failure should under no circumstances be aroused, for a person under its influence will not cope with difficulty in case he/she makes mistakes. Failures should be considered as spurs to fresh effort (Burklen, 1985).

In addition, many students have further disabilities that accompany their visual impairments, such as cognitive impairments or learning disabilities. It is essential to know that visually impaired students differ in their abilities to use their vision. These individual differences affect the way the student obtains information and learns.

Summing up, visually impaired students need concrete educational experiences that offer them the opportunity to explore objects and their environment thoroughly, using senses other than sight, and to learn by doing.

It is worth emphasising that working with visually impaired students can be not only challenging, but immensely rewarding. In essence, cooperation with a student who is visually handicapped requires sensitivity to the unique ways in which he or she is able to gain access to information.

1.4.1. The cohesion of skills – dual language linkage system

The linguistic skills layer is divided into receptive and productive (Harmer, 2004). I found the issue of the cohesion of productive and receptive skills within dual language linkage system crucial to analyse within the process of teaching-learning English as a foreign language to the visually impaired. Dual language linkage system is based upon two areas: skills and sensory intelligence, which incorporate audible, haptic and kinaesthetic intelligences (Gardner, 1993). Sensory intelligence absorbs sensory compensation that exists in three fields: echolocation, which stands for recognition of objects and physical environment by hearing perception, then kinaesthetic intelligence and haptic intelligence operated by touch experience (tactile perception).

The PLT process questions the division of skills into productive – writing and speaking – and receptive – listening and reading – in relation to visually handicapped students. Receptive skills turn to the productive layer. The exchange of skills is caused by visual impairment and the necessity of the usage of sensory compensation techniques involved in the PLT. In this dissertation I analyse receptive skills as productive ones through one dominant skill – speaking; reading and listening are directly connected with speaking comprehension. The PLT teaching-learning process focuses on the engagement of productive skills in the development of tactile awareness, which can also be seen as a supportive tool for transforming receptive skills into productive ones. Productive skills are enriched with tactile skills: on the one hand, they are skills themselves, and on the other, means to achieve skills. Parallel reading and dicto-listening are the modules that practise reading and listening through speaking comprehension (Figure 1).

Figure 1. The author's dual language linkage system

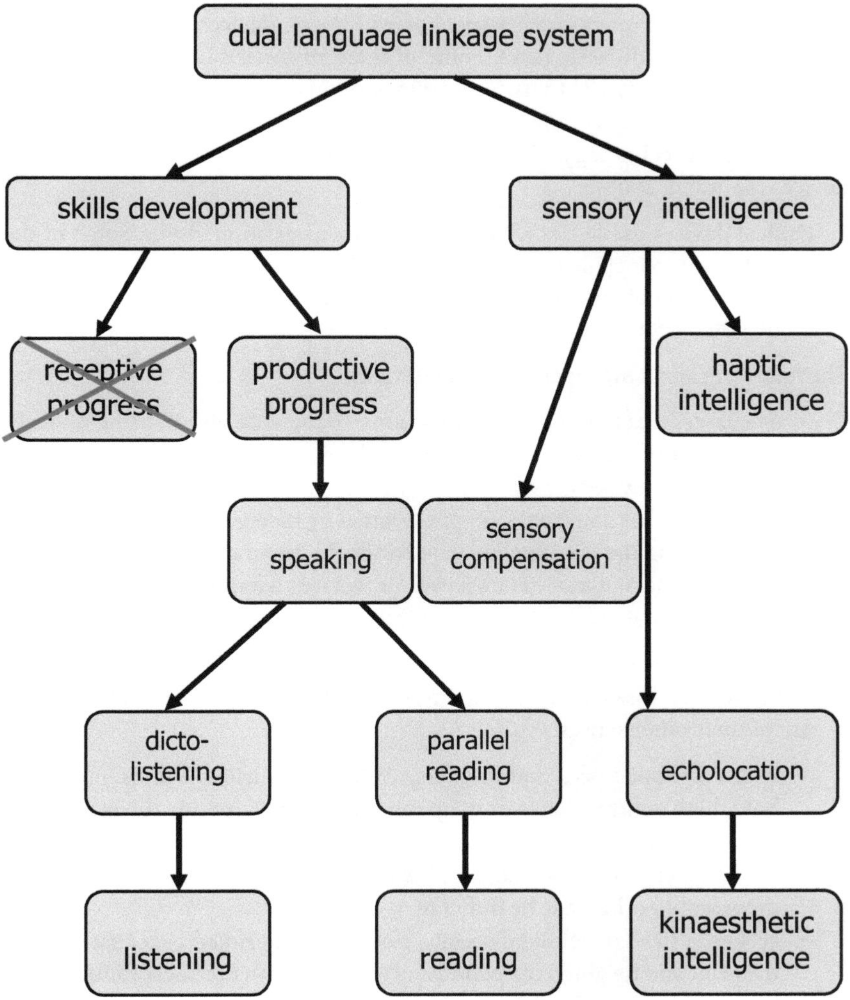

1.4.2. Special didactic devices for the visually impaired

Visually impaired students use a variety of equipment, devices, and tools to assist them with various didactic tasks. Some of them may need only a few adaptive devices, while others need to use several in combination.

These devices are generally categorised as optical devices, non-optical devices, and assistive technology. The following subchapter describes each category of devices (Spungin, 2008):

- Optical devices use lenses to optimise a person's existing vision. Some of the ways they do so include enlarging or modifying a visual image, altering the apparent position of an object, controlling light, and changing the apparent size of the visual field.

The following are some types of optical devices:

- ➢ eyeglasses that have two basic functions: to improve vision, using bifocals, prism lenses, contact lenses, and to reduce glare or excess light, both indoors and outdoors;
- ➢ magnifiers that make objects appear larger by increasing the size of the image reaching the eye; they may be handheld, mounted in a stand that sits on top of the material to be viewed, or worn as a loupe over eyeglasses;
- ➢ telescopes that are used to view objects at a distance.

- Non-optical devices are also utilised to assist visually impaired people to perform everyday tasks, to make maximum use of their sight and to enhance the use of their other senses.

    - ➢ wide felt-tipped pens and markers, available in various widths, produce a bold, high contrast letter or diagram; they usually provide the most effective contrast in black, but the use of different-coloured markers may help a student emphasise sections of his or her notes when scanning through them would otherwise be difficult;
    - ➢ acetate, a sheet of coloured acetate, placed over a printed page that darkens the print and heighten the contrast of the print with the background paper;
    - ➢ lamps with adjustable arms and controls to vary the intensity of light can provide the additional or dimmed illumination that a visually impaired student may require;

- large-print books and materials for students with low vision; the quality and size of the print, the typeface, and the spacing between letters and lines are all important considerations for legibility;
- bold-line paper, for students who find it difficult to see the lines on regular writing paper; the amount of white space between the lines can also vary to accommodate larger printing by a student with low vision;
- line markers and reading windows can be placed over print to isolate a single line or word; it may be especially helpful to students who find it difficult to focus on a word or to track a line of print;
- sun-visors and other shields; students who are light sensitive need to block out some of the light and glare around them; a hat or visor may also help reduce glare and visual discomfort;
- book stands are designed specifically for people with low vision; they help reduce postural fatigue by bringing the work closer to the reader's eyes.

Devices for enhancing tactile functioning (Czerwińska, 2008), (Piskorska et al., 2008):

- tactile graphics – graphic images, such as pictures, graphs, charts, maps that students are not able to see, are available and can be made into tactile formats that they can explore with their fingers;
- raised marks – special markers, adhesive-backed materials, and glues that leave raised marks that may be utilised to create lines or dots that can be easily felt;
- raised-line paper, on which lines are embossed to allow students to feel the lines;
- raised-line drawing boards – a rubber-covered board on which a sheet of acetate is placed; when someone draws or writes on the acetate with a pen or other pointed object, it produces raised lines that can be felt;
- teacher-made materials that provide visually impaired students with a rich source of unique tactile experiences that can enhance learning through touch and offer an opportunity for teachers to be creative.

Using devices that are equipped with sound can provide visually impaired students with access to information. Such devices may be either everyday equipment or specialised products for people with visual impairments.

Devices for enhancing auditory functioning (Spungin, 2008):

- talking books or recorded books,
- voice organisers and recorders – a variety of available recording devices can be used to record short notes that can be played at a later time,
- additional auditory devices – like talking watches, alarm clocks, money and colour identifiers.

The awareness and use of available special didactic devices in the PLT process lead to a noticeable development of communicative skills for the visually impaired, diminishing their physical and intellectual barriers.

Chapter Two: Concepts of mental therapy

2.0. Introductory remarks

Chapter three depicts emotions, personality and intelligence as enormously complex subjects to analyse with an emphasis put on axiological issues. Various personality theories have been presented: trait, psychoanalytic, behavioural, social learning, and humanistic, supporting Maslow's theory of needs. The central issue is covered by emotions that are not only related to intelligence, but are also subject to creative change. In other words, behind the trichotomy of intelligence, emotions, and creativity, there lies a unity – each shares features with others. Next, the area of motivation and flow appears in correlation with emotions, personality, and intelligence issues.

In my thesis, Gardner's intelligence structure exists in cohesion with the source of motivation that leads to self-esteem development of the students. The concept that will be discussed – so pivotal to this dissertation – is group therapy, developed through mental-haptic channels of the sandtray therapy, the Brain Linkage Method and the edu-kinaesthetic field.

2.1. Correlations between emotions and values

Cacioppo (Cacioppo et al., 2001:173) wrote that "emotions guide, enrich and ennoble life: they provide meaning to everyday existence: they render the valuation placed on life and property". Values shape emotions.

"Axiology is a branch of knowledge dealing with values" (Krzeszowski, 1997:22). According to Wierzbicka (Nowakowska-Kempna, 1995), axiological distinctions can be made within the good/bad dichotomy.

Values are results of human cognitive processes and the process of conceptualisation. The verb *to value* can be analysed within two senses (Krzeszowski, 1997): to estimate and to imply positive values attributed to valuable objects. Such attributing will be called valuation.

"Values are often confused with objects of value (valuable objects)… It is necessary to distinguish values as such from things to which values are attributed. Such things will be called bearers of values or briefly bearers" (Krzeszowski, 1997:22). Every bearer (thing) is an entity but not all entities can be called things. Krzeszowski (1997:23) explains the relation between values, objects of values, and people – "producers" of valuation: "Whatever values are attributed to various objects, these values are not inherent in the objects themselves but are attributed to these objects by people who conceive these objects as having a certain value". Values exist only in the phenomenological domain.

Values are the primary tool for maintaining fulfilment and satisfaction in life. They are also the primary tool for gaining control over a life that feels out of control (or feels like it may become so at any time). Unlike emotions, which change rapidly and are influenced by perceptions, values are the foundation of stability in a person's life. They remain relatively consistent throughout the course of life in adults. We all experience values or what we consider to have positive or negative value – all of us. No matter how neglected or diminished a role they can play in our lives, they exist just the same. Emotions are based on values. Without a foundation of values, value-based emotions cannot exist. Without value-based emotions, value-based decisions cannot be made. Each value has "the ability" to produce emotions: positive or negative. Our ability to comfort ourselves and provide emotional stability comes from our ability to manage our emotions. Our ability to manage our emotions comes from our ability to understand and commit to our values. This is imperative because without a base of values, we are destined to manage our lives through spontaneous, chaotic, behaviour-based emotions with little regard for long-term fulfilment. Value-based emotions are in a foundational commitment to long-term growth and life management. Value-based emotions promote stability, important to establish an individual's identity. Such emotions are consistent and stable.

Emotions have values as their formal objects. Values figure in the conditions for correctness of emotions but are not represented by emotions. Although emotions do not themselves represent or present values, they are nevertheless associated with some sort of intentional relation to values. Emotions should therefore be described as reactions to values or to what seems to be objects of values. In essence, values figure in the conditions of emotions and emotions are reactions to the felt value of objects and situations.

A few remarks should be made concerning the nature and strength of the associations between emotions and values. First of all, it should be noted that principle relations between values and emotions are reciprocal and we make no assumption concerning the direction of causation. Correlations may arise because behaviour directed by a particular type of value likely results in the experience of a particular emotion. On the other hand, frequent experience of a particular emotion will investigate behaviour from which people, for instance through self-perception, deduce that certain values are important to them. Second, unique correspondence of an emotion with a particular value type is unlikely because:

(a) mutual associations already exist between emotions and between values separately,
(b) emotions specify goals at a more abstract level, which may involve multiple, more specific goals as expressed by different values.

Summing up, values and emotions, in spite of their apparent correspondence in terms of goals, are different psychological constructs, specifying goals at a different level. Particularly, values express goals at a more specific level than the goals usually associated with emotions. Both constructs also relate to different psychological processes that need not necessarily coincide. Emotions can also arise, however, in situations that do not pertain to value conflicts. For example, I may get angry when I miss my bus, though missing the bus does not conflict with any value that I consider important. It should be noted that value importance can be related to differences in intensity of emotional experience.

Emotions provide common currency for values, values serve to choose motivations, and motivations prime actions.

The correlations between axiology and language are presented in subchapter 3.1.

2.2. Emotion, feeling, affect

Although the concept of emotion appears to be generally understood, it is surprisingly difficult to come up with a solid definition. When surveying emotion research in psychology, it is visible that various traditions hold different views on defining, studying and explaining emotions. Psychologists have offered a variety of definitions, each focusing on different manifestations or components of emotions.

There is no empirical solution to the debate on which component is sufficient or necessary to define emotions. There are various perspectives to understanding emotions. Emotion theory has its origins in philosophy (Strongman, 1996). Plato saw emotion as something which confounds, interrupts, gets in the way of or otherwise detracts from human reason. Solomon argues that Plato placed emotion somewhere between spirit and appetite, but it is clear that he viewed it as base. For Aristotle emotions were much more interesting facets of existence. He viewed them as being accounted for by a mixture of higher cognitive life and a lower sensual life. He saw emotions as being linked with pleasure and pain, and listed various specific emotions such as anger, fear and pity. Following Aristotle was Descartes' conceptualisation of emotions: his name being synonymous with dualism, Descartes had a place in emotion for physiological changes and behaviour as well as for mental processes such as perception, belief and memory. But the experience of emotion and hence its essence or core takes places in the soul.

The information about the world is carried to the soul via the pineal gland; the soul makes its deliberations and then sends messages back to the body, again via the pineal gland. After sending messages to the body, the soul then produces "a final mirror-image feeling of all that is going on" (Lyons, 1980:299). This is the emotion. Darwin had an important influence on the early understanding of emotion. He suggested that emotional expressions have not evolved, they do not depend on natural selection. Instead, he argued that they are either simply dependent on the way in which the nervous system is wired or possibly are remnants of old habits (Fridlund, 1992). McDougall's theory of emotions (1928) depended on some basic biological considerations and on an attempt to distinguish between emotions and feelings. He believed that the capacity to approach beneficial goals is fundamental to psychological functioning and that all behaviour stems from seeking food or from escaping or avoiding noxious stimuli. He argued that emotions occur as adjuncts to these basic processes, arising from the way in which we perceive the environment and various bodily changes. Although McDougall believed that just two feelings, pleasure and pain, modify all of our goal-directed behaviour, he also recognised the cognitive nature of human beings. This allows experiences to be fused and sets up unusual concentrations of feelings. He also implied that perception triggers emotion. According to McDougall, feelings depend on cognitions, whereas emotions are independent of cognition.

Then Ryle (1948) suggested that emotions are made of inclinations (motives), moods, agitations (or commotions) and feelings. The first three are propensities, not occurrences in the same way that feelings are. Papez's (1937) theory of emotion depended on the simple view that emotions imply behaviour (expression) and feelings (experience, subjective aspects). For Duffy (1962), emotion is a scientific concept, "worse than useless". She hypothesised that states of emotions must involve changes in energy level that are dependent on the stimulus. In this context, emotion simply represents an extreme of motivation or energy. Denzin (1984) provided the analysis of emotion from a phenomenological perspective – emotion is a form of consciousness, lived and experienced. "Emotion is self-feeling. Emotions are temporarily embodied, situated self-feelings that arise from emotional and cognitive social acts that people direct to self or have directed toward them by others" (p. 49). Rosaldo (1980) highlighted the interconnectedness of feelings, thoughts, and bodily reactions in the experience of emotions. Emotions are perceived by the mind, experienced in palpable bodily reactions, and felt as interior sensations called feelings. Plutchik (1980) defined emotion as an inferred, complex sequence of reactions, including cognitive evaluation, subjective change, and autonomic and neural arousal impulses to action. For him, emotion is multidimensional with dimensions of intensity, similarity and polarity. Any emotion can vary in intensity, or in its similarity to any other emotion; all emotions are polar. Plutchik (1980) discussed the importance of the language used in any analysis of emotion. He regarded subjective feelings as sufficient for emotion, but not as necessary; a person may have an emotion but remain unaware of it. From his perspective, emotion has two functions:

(1) to communicate information about intentions or probable behaviour,
(2) to increase the chances of survival when faced with emergencies.

Emotion can be modified by learning and can be seen as a form of behavioural homeostasis.

Siminov's (1970) theory of emotion begins with a definition of negative emotion: emotion equals need multiplied by the difference between the necessary information and the available information: $E = -N\ (In - Ia)$. Here, information refers to the possibility of reaching a goal due to a particular communication. If an organism cannot organise itself appropriately because there is a lack of information, the nervous system mechanism leading to negative emotions starts to act. Siminov saw positive emotion similarly. If an organism's needs are satisfied it is emotionally quiescent, but a surplus of information over what is necessary for satisfaction leads to positive emotions. Such positive emotions endure as do negative emotions and may facilitate behaviour. In Bower's view (Strongman, 1996), emotions are centrally placed in a network of meaning, and are connected to everything relevant, from related ideas, autonomic activity, muscular patterns, expressive patterns and events. Emotion matters are encoded propositionally with relevant events taking the form of subject-response-object. Izard (1991) viewed emotion as a motivational system, a process of personality which gives meaning to human existence and which determines behaviours. These are the ten fundamental emotions: interest, enjoyment, surprise, sadness, anger, disgust, contempt, fear, shame and shyness. All emotions have elements in common. They are non-cyclical, have unlimited generality and flexibility as motivators, and influence drives and other personality subsystems. According to his Differential Emotions Theory (DET), emotions are innate, are discrete from one another and each emotion is believed to be packaged with a specific and distinctive set of bodily and facial reactions. Davitz (1969) suggested that the meaning of various emotions depended on experience, and argued that this should be studied through language. From his standpoint,

(1) emotion is partly concerned with private, experienced events,
(2) the language of emotion reflects experiences but is also directly affected by linguistic considerations; people make mistakes in their descriptions of emotion and, in fact, learn to label the emotion from the situation,
(3) labelling emotion depends on experience; any change in experience will change the label and the state.

It is indisputable that emotions are a multifaceted phenomenon consisting of the following components (Strongman, 1996):

(1) cognitive reactions – perception, thinking and memory are involved in emotional expression,
(2) affect – all emotions are affective, involving a positive or negative state,
(3) physiological reactions – hormones are attributed to emotional states,
(4) behavioural responses – emotions motivate individuals to express feelings.

Summing up, emotions are whole-body phenomena that involve loosely-coupled changes in the domains of subjective experience, behaviour, and the central and peripheral physiology (Gross, 2009). Emotions have three primary functions: adaptation and survival, regulation, and communication. These three core features of emotion constitute the modal model of emotion: a person-situation transaction that compels attention, has particular meaning to an individual, and gives rise to a coordinated yet flexible multisystem response to the on-going person-situation transaction (Figure 2). The emotional responses generated by appraisals are thought to involve changes in experiential, behavioural, and neurobiological response systems (Gross, 2009).

Figure 2. The "modal model" of emotion

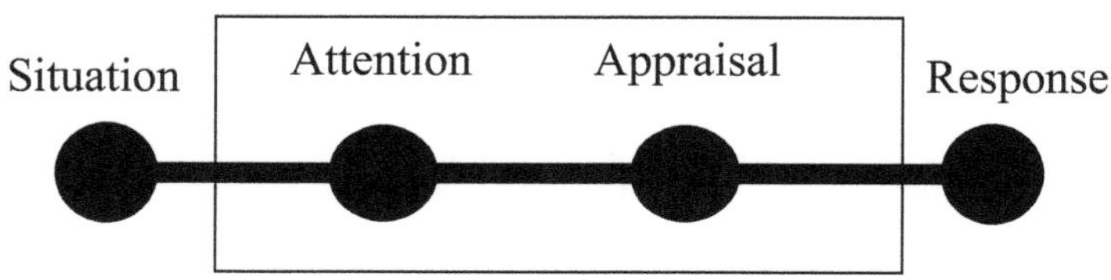

Most researchers today do not believe that *feelings*, *emotions*, and *affects* are the same notions. Feelings are only one aspect of emotional processes. The subjective aspect of emotion is, of course, so tightly bound up with the terms that emotion and feeling are often used interchangeably. But emotions not only make us feel something, they make us feel like doing something (Frijda, 1986). Following Scherer (Lyons, 1980), affect is used as the superordinate category for various kinds of states that involve relatively quick good-bad discriminations. Affect is used to refer to the experiential or behavioural components of emotions (Gross, 2009).

Although feeling and affect are routinely used interchangeably, it is important not to confuse affect with feelings and emotions. Affect is a pre-personal intensity corresponding to the passage from one experiential state of the body to another, implying an augmentation or diminution in that body's capacity to act. In Massumi's definition (Shouse, 2005), affect is not a personal feeling. Feelings are personal and biographical, emotions are social, and affects are pre-personal. A feeling is a sensation that has been checked against previous experiences and labelled. According to Wierzbicka (1971:30), "feeling is something that is felt, not experienced in words. Thoughts can be written in words but feelings cannot". An emotion is the projection/display of a feeling. An affect is a non-conscious experience of intensity; it is a moment of unformed and unstructured potential. Of the three central terms, affect is the most abstract because affect cannot be fully realised in language and is always prior to and/or outside of consciousness. Affect is the body's way of preparing itself for action in a given circumstance, by adding a quantitative dimension of intensity to the quality of an experience.

> Affects are comprised of correlated sets of responses involving the facial muscles, the viscera, the respiratory system, the skeleton, autonomic blood flow changes, and vocalizations that act together to produce an analogue of the particular gradient or intensity of stimulation impinging on the organism (Demos, 1995:19).

Affects, however, remain non-conscious and unformed and "are aroused easily by factors over which the individual has little control" (Demos, 1995:54). Without affects, feelings do not "feel" because they have no intensity, and without feelings rational decision-making becomes problematic (Shouse, 2005). The power of affect lies in the fact that it is unformed and unstructured (abstract). It is affect's "abstractivity" that makes it transmittable in ways that feelings and emotions are not, and it is because affect is transmittable that it is potentially such a powerful social force.

2.3. Measuring the intensity of emotions

In Brehm's view:

> Emotions are motivational states with the special function of producing adaptation to situational conditions. The emotional system lies in the central nervous system, that it is fast to react, able to change quickly from one emotional state to another, produces only one emotion at a time, and the *intensity* of that emotion is a nonmonotonic function of deterrence to the aim of the emotion (1999:2).

One of the most noticeable aspects of an emotion is its intensity. Emotions vary in intensity. There are many parameters that can be related to emotional intensity. These are various dimensions of the intensity of emotions (Sonnemans and Frijda, 1994):

(1) duration of the emotion and delay of its onset and peak,
(2) perceived bodily changes and strength of felt passivity,
(3) recollection and re-experience of the emotion,
(4) strength and severity of action tendency and severity of actual behaviour,
(5) belief changes and influence upon long-term behaviour,
(6) overall felt intensity.

Most specific dimensions correlated moderately with overall felt intensity. Special attention is given to the relation between the intensity and the duration of emotion.

It is problematic how the intensity of emotions should be operationalised or measured. Of course, the intensity of subjective feelings can be found as the criterion. Emotions can be felt to be intense for different reasons: causing an experience that would be called intense, and an intense personal feeling. The two kinds of intensity would not seem to be comparable, or meaningfully ranked on the same scale. This emphasises that subjective emotional intensity is not truly one-dimentional but multidimentional (Sonnemans and Frijda, 1994). Emotions are multicomponential phenomena that consist of momentary states, but also processes that stretch out over time. The major components are: affect (the feeling of pleasantness or unpleasantness), appraisal (the awareness of the meaning of the emotional event), state of action readiness, and behaviour; additional components include cognitive tunings and belief changes. Each component may vary more or less independently in magnitude and duration. This applies to the objective components, such as expressive behaviour, action readiness, and physiological response, and to the subjective components, such as affect, appraisal, belief changes, and one's awareness of the objective components.

Also, emotions have consequences that reflect the magnitude of impact of the eliciting event, and that might (or might not) influence the individual's estimate of the intensity of his/her emotion, such as later recurrence of the event in thought, influence upon one's conduct of life, and the formation of long-term goals. Emotion duration, of course, is an important aspect of emotion that also varies in magnitude.

Emotional intensity can be expressed in many different ways (Piechowski, 1991):

- positive feelings, negative feelings, both positive and negative feelings,
- bodily symptoms such as tense stomach, sinking heart, blushing, headache, nausea,
- inhibition – timidity and shyness,
- strong affective memory,
- fears and anxieties,
- depressive moods,
- emotional ties and attachments to others,
- critical self-evaluation and self-judgment, feelings of inadequacy and inferiority.

Emotions are internal affective states; only their outward expression, physiological reactions and bodily responses can be measured. Each instrument that is claimed to measure emotions in fact measures one of the components of emotions. There are an abundant number of instruments and great diversity in approaches to measure emotions. Today's instruments range from simple pen-and-paper scales to dazzling high-tech equipment that measures brain waves or eye movements.

A distinction can be also made between non-verbal and verbal instruments (Brehm, 1999):

(1) Non-verbal instruments

This category comprises instruments that measure expressive or physiological components. An expressive reaction is the facial, vocal, and postural expression that accompanies emotions. Instruments that measure this component of emotion fall into two major categories: those measuring facial and those measuring vocal expressions. Facial expression instruments are based on theories that link expression features to distinct emotions. Examples of such theories are the Facial Action Coding System (Shouse, 2005), and the Maximally Discriminative Facial Moving Coding System (Izard, 1991). Also subtle expressions, invisible to the naked eye, can be measured because the facial muscle activity of these expressions result in electrical potentials. Like the facial expression instruments, vocal instruments are based on theories that link patterns of vocal cues to emotions (Gross, 2009). These instruments measure the effects of emotion in multiple vocal cues such as average pitch, pitch changes, intensity colour, speaking rate, voice quality or articulation.

A physiological reaction (activation or arousal, e.g. increases in heart rate) is the change in activity in the autonomic nervous system that accompanies emotions. Emotions show a variety of physiological manifestations that can be measured with a diverse array of techniques. Examples of instruments include those that measure blood pressure responses, skin responses, papillary responses, brain waves, and heart responses.

The major advantage of non-verbal instruments is that, as they are language-independent, they can be used in different cultures. A second advantage is that they are unobtrusive because they do not disturb participants during the measurement. In addition, these instruments are often claimed to be less subjective than self-reporting instruments because they do not rely on the participants' own assessment of the emotional experience. This class of instruments has several limitations. First, these instruments can only reliably assess a limited set of basic emotions such as anger, fear, or surprise. Moreover, these instruments cannot assess mixed emotions.

(2) Verbal instruments

Verbal instruments assess the subjective feeling component of emotions; subjective feeling (e.g. feeling happy or inspired) is the conscious awareness of the emotional state. Each emotion involves a specific feeling which is a basic, irreducible kind of mental element (Lyons, 1980). These subjective feelings can only be measured through self-reporting. The most often used self-reporting instruments require respondents to report their emotions with the use of a set of rating scales or verbal protocols.

Two major advantages of verbal instruments are that rating scales can be assembled to represent any set of emotions, and can be used to measure mixed emotions.

In my view, a simple, well-organised verbal instrument such as *The Positive and Negative Affect Schedule (PANAS questionnaire)* implemented during the psycho-linguistic therapy "Touching the World" enables the measuring of emotional responses – the intensity of positive and negative affects.

Affects comprise both positive and negative dimensions and are complex chains of events triggered, understood, revealed or released by a certain stimulus – such as the PLT. The PANAS (Watson et al., 1988) is a lexical measure developed in the North American setting. The 20-item PANAS covers two mood scales (Figures 3 and 4), one measuring positive affects (10 items – excited, alert, interested, strong, enthusiastic, proud, inspired, determined, attentive, and active), and the other measuring negative affects, using such adjectives as distressed, upset, guilty, scared, hostile, irritable, ashamed, nervous, jittery, afraid. Each mood item is related to a definite number and is rated on a 5-point Likert scale, ranging from 1 – very slightly or not at all, through 2 – a little, 3 – moderately, 4 – quite a bit, to 5 – extremely, to indicate the extent to which the respondent felt that way in the indicated time frame. The authors (Watson et al., 1988) used the scale to measure affect at this moment, the past few months, the past year, and generally (on average).

Negative affect (NA) and positive affect (PA) reflect dispositional dimensions, with high NA epitomised by subjective distress and unpleasant engagement, and low NA by the absence of these feelings. By contrast, PA represents the extent to which an individual experiences pleasurable engagement with the environment. Thus, emotions such as enthusiasm and alertness are indicative of high PA, whilst lethargy and sadness characterise low PA. Watson et al. (1988) point out that PA and NA are predominantly defined by the activation of positive and negative affects (i.e. the lower ends of each dimension are typified by its absence). Thus, to emphasise the activated nature of each of these constructs, it was argued that positive affect and negative affect should be renamed positive activation and negative activation, respectively. In the present work, these labels are to be regarded as interchangeable.

However, there are many problems with these measures. Before one can measure emotions, one must be able to characterise emotions and distinguish them from other states. It is important to note that questionnaires measure what people say they feel and not what they feel.

Figure 3. Positive affects

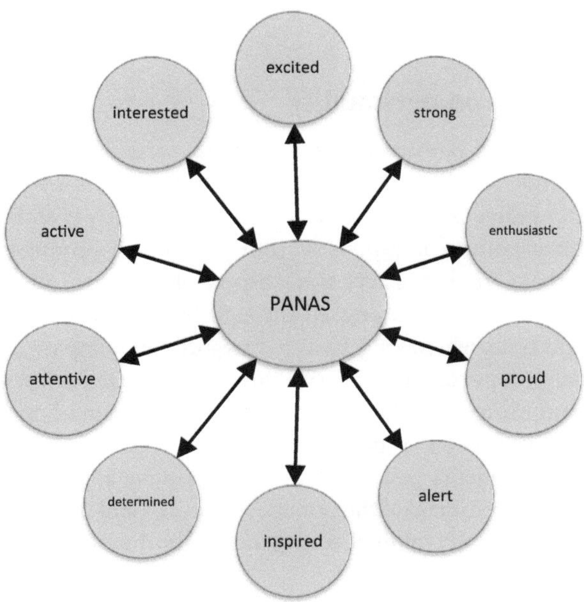

Figure 4. Negative affects

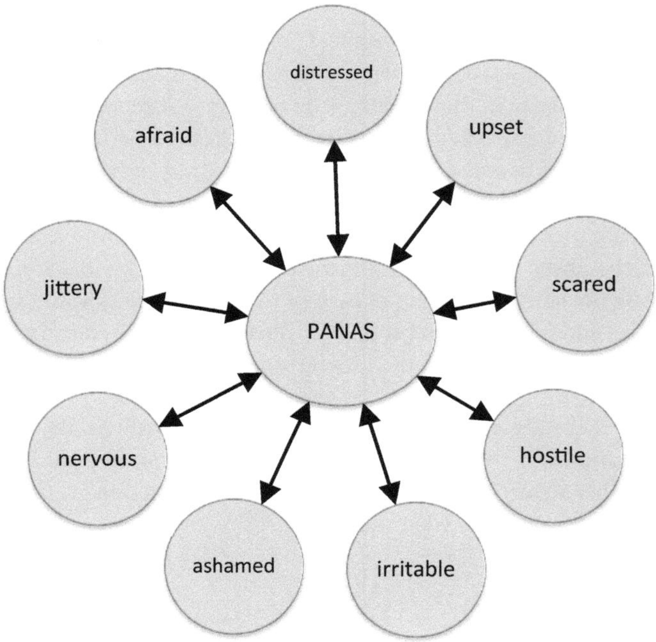

2.4. Perspectives on personality

A proper definition of personality usually makes certain points: personality is a reflection of individual uniqueness. That is, personality is a sort of collective term relating to individual distinctive qualities. Personality is an internal, mental, and emotional pattern of response to the environment – a pattern of thought, feeling, and behaviour that affects every aspect of a person's life (Gatchel and Mears, 1982). Personality is expressed through the aspect of individual differences: types and traits which are a basis to categorise or compare individuals.

I examine diverse personality theories such as *biological, trait, psychodynamic, behaviourist* and *existential* that I found crucial in understanding personality; I considered various aspects of personality perspectives to help myself and my visually impaired students with an increase in positive affects and decrease in negative ones. The awareness of them made us (myself and my students), I hope, linguistically and mentally fulfilled during the psycho-linguistic therapy "Touching the World".

The following perspectives are taken into consideration:

The biological perspective

Biological models of personality (Engler, 1985) suggest that anatomical and biochemical factors are the primary determinants of personality style and behaviour. In general, there are the following broad biological models:

1. the body-type model holding that temperament and personality are tied to body structures;
2. the genetic model emphasising that personality and behaviour have strong genetic components; it argues that because obvious physical features are quite similar among close relatives, personality and behaviour should be similar as well;
3. the neuroanatomical model holding that personality and behaviour are strongly controlled by neuroanatomical structures; therefore, just as individuals differ with regard to obvious external features (such as height or weight), they should differ in the functioning of various brain areas;
4. the biochemical model arguing that brain chemicals, especially the neurotransmitters that pass nerve signals from a nerve cell to a nerve cell, exert strong control over behaviour and personality and, further, that the amounts of these substances differ widely among individuals. This variation in the amounts of chemicals may thus account for personality differences.

While there is some evidence to support various biological models, even most of their proponents recognise that environment may modify or change some biological factors. Moreover, biological research into personality suffers from extensive methodological problems. It is often not possible to determine whether a biochemical substance causes a given behaviour (such as depression), or whether the behaviour causes a biochemical change.

The trait perspective

Trait theory has much in common with the biological perspective, since both assume the existence of stable, internal dispositions that affect behaviour. Trait theorists (Arndt, 1974) assume that personality is determined by enduring dispositions or traits. They hold that individuals can be described best by referring to clusters of measurable traits that they possess. Indeed, they say that individuals differ because of the degree to which they express various traits. Trait theory is closely akin to the dispositional attributional theory, an approach that explains a person's actions or personality by attributing them to some stable, internal disposition such as an attitude, habit, or motive. Allport (Murray, 1938) assumes that traits are real neuropsychic structures that determine behaviour. They are hierarchically organised into a meaningful whole or personality. Cattell advances a theory that is similar to Allport's in its view of human personality as a hierarchically organised system of traits (Engler, 1985).

Trait theorists hold that traits alone are sufficient to explain behaviour. Other personality psychologists believe traits to be completely irrelevant. The truth seems to lie somewhere between these two extremes. To predict and understand behaviour, researchers must assess both people's personalities and their current situations or environments.

The psychodynamic perspective

While biological theories (Arndt, 1974) speak of concrete, physical factors such as the brain or bio-chemicals as personality determinants, the psychodynamic perspective includes mental or psychological factors. Indeed, psychodynamics means mental energies. The best illustration of a psychodynamic factor is the unconscious mind, which plays a prominent role in many psychodynamic personality theories.

Although there are many types of psychodynamic personality theories, psychoanalysis being perhaps the best example, they all share several features:

- ✓ Behaviour or personality is influenced chiefly by early childhood experience.
- ✓ Personality is often hidden or camouflaged by a veneer of outer responses, an assumption that rests on the primacy of the unconscious mind.

The following list summarises the chief assumptions of some of the major psychodynamic approaches (Murphy, 1966):

- ➢ Classical psychoanalysis that is associated with Freud, who argued that humans must pass through determined psychosexual stages and that the frustration of steps within these stages shapes personality. Sexual and aggressive drives are the principal motivators of behaviour.
- ➢ Ego psychology that is related to Hartmann and Erikson. This model does not assume that humans are motivated principally by sexual and aggressive drives, nor does it hold that conflict is certain. The ego is the major personality agent that seeks to adapt behaviour to the external environment.
- ➢ Neo-Freudian theories that include those of Adler, Jung, and Sullivan. Their models place much more emphasis on adaption to society that did Freudian psychology and give much greater attention to interpersonal communication and feelings of insecurity.

- Transactional analysis is associated with Berne. This model of personality blends Freudian and neo-Freudian psychologies and has its own special language. Personality is thought to be determined early in life by parent-child relationships. Instincts and genetics play minimal roles.

The social learning perspective – behaviourist model

The psychologist John Watson (Maddi, 1976) argued that psychologists should be interested only in what is observable and hence objective. He insisted that the notions of personality, mind, self, and consciousness were not matters of concern for the science of psychology. The only source of direct data, he said, is overt behaviour. Behaviourism therefore focused chiefly on observable actions. Initially, Watson and other radical behaviourists (Murray, 1938) concentrated primarily on how behaviour was acquired. They rejected mental constructs such as personality to explain behaviour. They held that the psychoanalytic phenomenon of repression, in which certain thoughts or feelings are kept from conscious awareness, could be explained as learning to forget in order not to deal with unpleasant material. This change owed a great deal to Miller and Dollard, who reinterpreted many psychoanalytic terms within the framework of learning theory. It is quite common for learning theorists to speak of internal processes. Even the radical behaviourist Skinner (1974) acknowledged the existence of personality, although he attributed its existence to environmental reinforcement.

In the 1980s the trend was towards emphasis on the interaction of phenomenological, biological, and learning factors. This approach, known as cognitive social learning, holds basically that behaviour is a result of multiple factors. It maintains that three classes of factors contribute to personality development: current social and environmental conditions, the biochemical-neurological state of the individual, and the psychological or cognitive state of the individual. This model argues that humans learn in complex ways that involve past experience, expectations, current thoughts, feelings, social context and neurological processes. Personality is thus a function of many variables.

The following issues summarise major behaviourist assumptions (Engler, 1985):

- Radical behaviourism, which is associated with Watson and Skinner, says that all behaviour, including personality, is learned. This approach emphasises the importance of dealing with observable behaviour rather than with inner dispositions or traits.
- Psychodynamic learning, which is related to Dollard and Miller, interprets some basic Freudian ideas in terms of learning principles and the methods of

experimental laboratory research on behaviour. Again, the major assumption is that all behaviour is learned.

- Cognitive social learning, which is connected with Rotter, Bandura, and Mischel, is like radical behaviourism in that it emphasises the importance of dealing with observable behaviour and situational factors in learning. However, it also takes into account a person's unique biological and psychological characteristics.

Kazdin (1980) summarises the behavioural approach as a departure from the traditional conception of behaviour by rejecting inferred motives, hypothesised needs, impulses, and drives which supposedly explain behaviour. The emphasis is placed upon environmental, situational, and social determinants that influence behaviour.

The phenomenological-existential perspective

The phenomenological-existential perspective resembles the psychodynamic approach more than it does the biological one, for it suggests that personality is largely determined by the individual's unique perception of reality. These theorists focus on what it feels like to be human, not upon why we are human. They usually speak of internal mental processes, but not anatomical, biochemical, or environmental forces.

Maslow (1970) assumes that human beings have an inborn drive pushing them towards actualisation of their potential. This model also argues for the existence of a hierarchy of needs. The guiding personality component is the perceptual agent, or the self. Rogers (Maddi, 1976) resembles Maslow both in assuming a push towards fulfilment and in formulating an internal structure called "the self". Rogers places more emphasis on internal conflicts, as opposed to Maslow's emphasis on satisfying specific hierarchical needs. Kelly depicts a model of personality that suggests that the individual formulates hypotheses (constructs) about future events and then tests them against reality. Personality, then, is a set of constructs aimed at anticipating future data.

The study of personality involves many aspects of human behaviour, ones I reconsidered for the proper analysis of the subject matter.

2.5. Maslow's pyramid of needs

"The link between visual impairments and motivation to learn foreign languages becomes obvious when one perceives the compensatory role that foreign languages perform in the lives of people with visual impairments" (Krzeszowski, 2012:36).

I focused on Maslow's theory in the PLT to highlight the correlation between needs, seen through visual impairment, personality perspectives, and finally motivation development of the visually impaired students.

Human beings need to fulfil various needs. Deficit or basic needs should be covered to cater to higher-being needs. In case of fulfilment of basic needs, such needs are no longer employed as a source of motivation. The structure of appearance of definite needs corresponds with people's personalities. Alderfer (Dunlop, 1977) emphasises that some needs exist in parallel. The degree of fulfilment influences the level of intensity of needs that shapes motivation. Maslow developed the hierarchy of needs model in the 1940s and 50s, and the hierarchy of needs theory remains valid today for understanding human motivation and personal development. Maslow (1970) thought extensively about what motivates people and developed a detailed, hierarchical list of needs that motivate people toward purposeful goals. The list includes two kinds of needs: basic needs (or deficiency needs) and growth needs (or being needs). He placed all human needs in a pyramidal arrangement to show that those needs at the bottom of the pyramid must be satisfied before those that are placed higher (Figure 5). He noticed that some human needs take precedence over others. Maslow laid out five broad layers: physiological needs, the needs for safety and security, the needs for love and belonging, the needs for esteem, and the need to actualise the self, in that order.

- Physiological needs are the ones people must satisfy before they can seek anything else in life. These include the needs for water, food, sleep and air. According to Maslow they drive behaviour.
- Safety and security needs. When the physiological needs are largely taken care of, this second layer of needs comes into consideration. People become increasingly interested in finding physical and psychological safety – safety ranks as the primary need for humans. They might develop the need for structure and order. Emotional safety appears in parallel with physical safety.
- Love and belonging needs. Physiological needs and safety needs lead people to fulfil psychological needs by developing affectionate relationships; until safety and security needs are satisfied, humans will not be primarily motivated by desires for love, affection, and belonging to a group or family. Maslow also believes that unsatisfied needs of love and belongingness warp the individual, stifling growth.
- Esteem needs. Maslow noted two versions of esteem needs, a lower one and a higher one. The lower one is the need for the respect of others, the need for status, fame, attention, appreciation dignity, even dominance. The higher form

involves the need for self-respect, including such feelings as confidence, competence, achievement, independence and freedom. The negative version of these needs leads to low self-esteem and inferiority complexes. Esteem needs motivate people to improve their positions in the world, and they represent the prelude to the highest possible need and motivational level, self-actualisation.

All of the preceding four levels he called deficit needs or D-needs (Figure 5).

Figure 5. Maslow's pyramid of needs

Being Needs

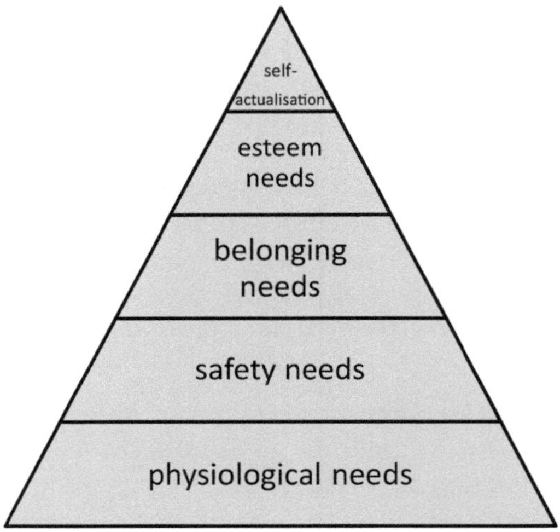

Deficit Needs

Maslow (1943) considers these levels also in terms of homeostasis. Homeostasis is the principle by which a furnace thermostat operates. In an analogous way, the human body – when it lacks a certain substance – develops a hunger for it. When the hunger is fulfilled, then it stops. Maslow simply extends the homeostatic principle to needs such as safety, belonging, and esteem. He emphasises all these needs as essentially survival needs. Even love and esteem are found crucial for the maintenance of health. He claims that these needs are built into people genetically, like instincts. He calls them instinctoid – instinct-like needs.

In terms of overall development human beings move through these levels. Under stressful conditions, or when survival is threatened, people can regress to a lower level of needs. If they experience significant problems along their development – a period of extreme insecurity or loss – they may "fixate" on that set of needs for the rest of their lives. This is Maslow's understanding of neurosis.

Maslow used a variety of terms to refer to the apex of the hierarchy. He called it growth motivation (in contrast to deficit motivation), being needs (or B-needs, in contrast to D-needs), and self-actualisation. These are the needs that do not involve balance and homeostasis. Once engaged, they continue to be felt. In fact, they are likely to become stronger as people "feed" them. They involve continuous desire to fulfil potentials. They are a matter of becoming the most complete, the fullest, "self" – hence the term self-actualisation.

The question becomes just what exactly does Maslow's self-actualisation mean? To answer that, the term called self-actualisers ought to be analysed. Maslow used a qualitative method called biographical analysis for explanation (Maslow 1970). He began by picking out a group of people – some historical figures, some people he had known – who he felt clearly met the standard of self-actualisation along with 12 unnamed people who were alive at the time Maslow did his research. He examined their biographies, writings, their deeds, and developed a list of qualities that seemed characteristic of those people. They were reality-centred, which means they could differentiate what is fake and dishonest from what is real and genuine. They were problem-centred, meaning they treated life's difficulties as problems demanding solutions, not as personal troubles to be railed at or surrendered to. And they had a diverse perception of means and ends. They felt that the ends do not necessarily justify the means, and the means could be ends themselves, and that the means – the journey – was often more important than the ends. The self-actualisers also had a different way of relating to others. First, they enjoyed solitude and were comfortable being alone. They enjoyed deeper personal relations with a few close friends and family members, rather than more shallow relationships with people. They enjoyed autonomy, relative independence from physical and social needs. And they resisted enculturation, that is, they were not susceptible to social pressure to be "well adjusted". They were, in fact, nonconformists in the best sense. They had a quality he called acceptance of self and others. On the other hand, they were strongly motivated to change negative qualities in themselves that could be changed. Along with this issue comes spontaneity and simplicity: they preferred being themselves rather than being pretentious or artificial. Further, they had a sense of humility and respect towards others that Maslow also called democratic values – meaning that they were open to ethnic and individual variety. They had a quality he called human kinship – social interest, compassion, humanity. And this was accompanied by a strong ethic that was spiritual, but seldom conventionally religious in nature. And those people had a certain freshness of appreciation, an ability to see things with wonder. Along with this appears the ability to be creative, inventive, and original. Finally, these people tended to have more peak experiences than an average person.

Maslow discovered several imperfections in self-actualisers. They often suffered considerable anxiety and guilt. Some of them were absent-minded and overly kind. And finally, some of them had unexpected moments of ruthlessness, surgical coldness. Two other points he makes about the self-actualisers: their values were natural and seemed to flow effortlessly from their personalities. They also appeared to transcend many of the dichotomies others accept as being undeniable, such as differences between the spiritual and the physical.

The idea of self-actualisation drives all creatures to various things that interfere with the "full" effectiveness of life force. If people are deprived of their basic physical needs, live under threatening circumstances, are isolated from others or have no confidence in their abilities, they may continue to survive, but it will not be as fulfilling a life as it could be. The paradox is: the more secure individuals feel about themselves, the more open and vulnerable they can be around others. The visually handicapped find themselves physically and emotionally insecure due to their impairment. The basic level of needs is not fulfilled. The loss of sight has its consequences in achieving goals of love and belonging or activating low self-esteem and inferiority complexes. They do not fully actualise their potentials.

In essence, the needs for safety and security are, as have been mentioned, basic needs, meaning that without their gratification the person will not thrive, much less be able to move onto higher motivational states. Meeting safety and security needs assures the individual of relative freedom from fear, anxiety and unpredictability.

2.6. Motivation and flow

Motivation is incorporated in the field of affective factors, influencing the learning process. The variety of definitions of motivation seems unending.

According to Freud (Murphy, 1966), the subconscious is a source of motivation. It includes the aspects that are not easily available to awareness, including drives, instincts, memories, and emotions associated with trauma or loss. Jung (1977) adds the part of the psyche that makes his theory stand out from all others: the collective subconscious that influences our experiences and behaviours (most especially emotional ones) and directs motivation. Adler (Pintrich and Schunk, 2002) postulates motivating force, called striving for perfection, behind all behaviour and experience. It implies a desire to fulfil potentials and come closer to the ideal. Another word that Adler used to refer to motivation was compensation. Personality could be accounted for by the ways people compensate or overcome their problems. His motivational aspect relates to Maslow's self-actualisation. Maslow (1970) coins the term metamotivation to describe the motivation of people who go beyond the scope of the basic needs and strive for constant betterment. Metamotivated people are driven by being needs, instead of deficiency needs. Skinner (Weiner, 1992) claims that an organism encounters a special kind of stimulus, naming motivation as a reinforcing stimulus. This special kind has the effect of increasing the operant – that is, the behaviour occurring just before the reinforcer. This is the operant conditioning: behaviour is followed by a consequence, and the nature of the consequence modifies the organism's tendency to repeat behaviour. Bandura (ibidem) depicts the learning process in diverse stages: attention, retention, reproduction and motivation. He distinguished three segments of motivation: past reinforcement, promised reinforcements (incentives that are in people's imagination), and vicarious reinforcement (seeing and recalling the model of being reinforced). He also pays attention to negative motivation, comparing it to punishment – past, promised and vicarious. Allport (Maddi, 1976) suggests that human behaviour is motivated by something functioning in a manner expressive of the self – which he called *propriate* functioning. Most of the things people are involved in during their lives are a matter of their being. *Propriate* comes from the word *proprium*, which in Allport's view stands for an essential concept of self. *Self* equals motivation "for self". The self itself covers the motivational layer, being the source of it. Snygg and Combs' (Pintrich and Schunk, 2002) understanding of motivation relates to the basic need of everyone, i.e., preserving and enhancing the phenomenal self. The phenomenal self is the person's own view of him- or herself. Learning is a matter of improving the quality of one's phenomenal field by extracting some detail from the confusion because that detail is meaningful to the person. May (Pintrich and Schunk, 2002) also turns his attention to motivation. His basic motivational construct is the *daimonic*, which is the entire system of motives, different for each individual. It is composed of a collection of specific motives called *daimons*. Basically, he says a *daimon* is anything that can take over the person. Lier (Pintrich and Schunk, 2002:98) in his attempt to distinguish the sources of motivation claims that there are three of them:

> Past, which consists of events, one has already experienced, present that includes current attitudes towards the activity, here flow plays a distinctive role; and finally, future sources of motivation that consist of instrumental and integrative actions that direct individuals' goals.

The motivation stimulus covers also the issue of extraversion-introversion as a salient factor of the motivational existence. Eysenck (Weiner, 1992) claims that extraversion-introversion is a matter of balance of inhibition and excitation in the brain itself. Excitation is the brain waking itself up, getting into an alert, learning state. Inhibition is the brain calming itself down, either in the usual sense of relaxing, or in the sense of protecting itself in the case of overwhelming stimulation. Intrinsic motivation, called self-motivation, refers to a highly desired form of incentive that stems from a person's internal desire for self-satisfaction or pleasure in performing the task itself. Malone and Lepper define this issue in terms of what people will do without external inducement. Among the factors that promote intrinsic motivation are challenge, curiosity, control, competition, cooperation, or recognition (it requires the process or the product of the activity to be visible) (Deci and Ryan, 2000). For Maslow, intrinsic motivation was definitely more powerful than extrinsic. As far as his hierarchy of needs is concerned, "we are ultimately motivated to achieve self-actualisation once the basic physical, safety and community needs are met. No matter what extrinsic rewards are present or absent, we will strive for self-esteem and fulfilment" (Brown and Vaughan, 2009:153). Ellis (Deci and Ryan, 2000) claims that extrinsic motivation may have a negative impact on individuals and rather interfere with intrinsic motivation. Also Crookes and Schmidt (Deci and Ryan, 2000) are in favour of intrinsic motivation, especially when long-term retention is taken into account. Intrinsic motivation is the prototype of autonomous activity; when people are intrinsically motivated, they are self-determined by definition (Raffini, 1996). Due to such feelings of autonomy and self-determination, intrinsically motivated individuals are expected to maintain their effort and engagement, even when no external rewards are offered. Deci and Ryan (2000) depict intrinsic motivation as voluntary and spontaneous, independent of reinforcement or biological drives, and needing no external reward. Van Lier (May, 1996) proposes two layers of intrinsic motivation: first, a basic, organismic motivation consisting of intentionality, affect and effort, and second, a specifically human motivation, grafted onto this organismic one, including consciousness and choice. Therefore, extrinsic motivation has traditionally been seen as something that undermines intrinsic motivation. Harter (cited in Williams and Burden, 1997:124) views intrinsic and extrinsic motivation as "opposite ends of a continuum". Therefore, Dornyei (Deci and Ryan, 2000) states that the environmental context (a teacher, atmosphere, methods, expectancies of success and failure), goals, the feeling of autonomy and self-efficacy, all significantly affect intrinsic motivation. They take part in the way that they promote persistence, enhance increased effort, and foster direct attention towards goal-relevant actions.

Motivational issues are organised in diverse categories of involvement (Pintrich and Schunk, 2002). First, there are biological motivations, mostly needs for air, water, or pleasure. Secondly, social motivations, which may build on biological motivations, especially instinct complexes, but which vary enormously depending on culture, individual social situations and learning. Social motivation includes the need for acceptance, attention or approval. Third, there are the more personal motivations that are based on the experiences of the individual, especially habits, defence mechanisms, and personality styles. Last but not least, higher motivations appear. These are conscious and are perceived by people, providing their lives with meaning. There seem to be two broad kinds: the first, competence motivation, includes motives such as the desire to learn, attain competence and mastery, even the desire to be creative. The second, altruistic motivation, includes Adler's social concern, compassion, and love (Raffini, 1996). Gardner (1972) labels motivation as a notion strongly connected with attitudes and beliefs towards learning a language. In Gardner's motivation theory the key issue is the relationship between motivation and orientation, which is his term for a goal. Gardner's theory is in favour of the premise that orientations are not part of motivation but function merely as motivational antecedents. According to Gardner, motivation comprises three components: motivational intensity, desire to learn the language, and attitudes towards learning the language. Thus, in this view motivation refers to a kind of central mental "engine" or "energy-centre" that comprises effort, will (cognition) and task-enjoyment (affect). Gardner claims that these three components intermingle, since a truly motivated individual displays all three. The role of orientations is to help arouse motivation and focus it towards a set of goals, either with a strong integrative quality, or a strong instrumental one. According to Andrejewski-Lewenstern, motivation in language learning can be broadly understood as the main motive power that arouses an organism to action towards a desired goal (Deci and Ryan, 2000). Dornyei (Pintrich and Schunk, 2002) identifies several factors which are influential and contribute to L2 motivation. He suggests that interest in foreign languages, cultures and people, desire to broaden one's view, desire for new stimuli and challenges as well, are crucial factors in L2 motivation. Schmidt expands this view with a notion of determination that is a key factor. Julkunen (Pintrich and Schunk, 2002) in his research claims that communicative orientation is as important as intrinsic motivation. He adds feelings of helplessness or anxiety as core elements of success or attitudes towards a teacher or teaching method. Motivation is no longer seen as a reflection of certain inner forces such as instincts, drives or needs, emotional states or psychical energy. Nor is it perceived strictly in terms of habit formation, as a function of stimuli and reinforcement, rather it is focused on thoughts, beliefs, feelings and other processes that are transformed into action.

Flow theory is closely associated with high motivation, and its deep level of fulfilment and involvement in totally effortless activity. Flow emphasises a feeling of satisfaction and enjoyment. The state of flow is placed "between boredom and anxiety and shows a harmonious proportion between the amount of challenge in activities and individual capabilities" (Pintrich and Schunk, 2002:284).

The term flow was used by Csikszentmihalyi (2008) to refer to an optimal state of mind in which an individual feels cognitively efficient, deeply involved, highly motivated and also experiences a high level of enjoyment. Csikszentmihalyi (1993) developed the term to describe the sense of total involvement; he defined flow experience as a situation in which people perceive themselves as having a high level of skills and are put with challenges that stretch these skills. Flow tends to exist when a person faces a clear set of goals that requires appropriate responses and appears when a person's skills are fully involved in overcoming a challenge that is just above manageable. Csikszentmihalyi claims that flow can be achieved if some conditions are fulfilled: people's minds and bodies must be completely involved. The rates of their concentration are very high; moreover they are not worried about failure, they lose an ordinary sense of self-conscious worry.

Flow theory states that intrinsic motivation in everyday life is a function of the skills that a person feels "to possess in relation with the activity and the perceived challenges of the activity" (Csikszentmihalyi, 1996:88). He claims that when challenges and skills are high and in relative balance with each other, an individual tends to experience flow in consciousness and intrinsic motivation is the highest. Intrinsic motivation is lower in all other combinations of levels of challenges and skills. Therefore, the experience of flow is strongly connected with intrinsic motivation (Csikszentmihalyi, 2008).

According to flow theory two types of personality exist: *autotelic* and *exotelic*. Individuals with autotelic personalities experience flow more often and devote more time to hobbies or work. Gradually growing challenges cause the autotelics' skills to tend to develop together with the feeling of growing satisfaction, self-esteem and interest. The exotelic personality is motivated by an outside goal. The autotelics' levels of perceived challenges and skills are more balanced than those of non-autotelics (exotelics).

On the basis of the following conditions, Csikszentmihalyi formulated the following dimensions: clear and distinct goals, immediate direct feedback, consolidation of individuals' actions and awareness, personal skills well suited to challenges, an authentic sense of potential control, a modified and distorted sense of time, concentration on a task at hand. People who experience flow also describe a sense of control over a situation or activity as essential.

2.7. Memory issues

Memory must also play an important role in language use. However, memory itself is not a unitary concept, because numerous different characteristics and processes seem to be involved in remembering.

I focus on memory notions due to the PLT repetition programme that emphasises the beginning and final effects of "memory structure", achieved in L2.

According to cognitive psychology, human behaviour rests upon a number of cognitive processes such as thinking, memory, perception and language processing.

Humans are limited-capacity processors. Shiffrin and Schneider (1977) conceived of the differences in the processing capacity necessary for various mental operations in a dichotomous way: either a task requires a relatively large amount of processing capacity, or it proceeds automatically and demands little processing energy. They conceived of memory as a large collection of nodes that become "complexly inter associated" through learning. Each node is a grouping or set of informational elements. Most of the nodes are inactive and passive and, when in this state, the interconnected system of nodes is called long-term store. When, because of some kind of external stimulus, a small number of these nodes is activated, the activated nodes constitute short-term store. There are two ways in which these nodes become activated: the automatic and the controlled modes of information processing. Automatic processing involves the activation of certain nodes in memory, every time the appropriate inputs are present. This activation is a learned response that has been built up through the consistent mapping of the same input to the same pattern of activation over many trials. Since an automatic process utilises a relatively permanent set of associative connections in long-term storage, most automatic processes require an appreciable amount of training to develop fully. Once learned, an automatic process occurs rapidly and is difficult to suppress or alter. The second node of information processing, controlled processing, is not a learned response, but a temporary activation of nodes in a sequence. This activation is under attentive control of the subject and, since attention is required, only one such sequence can normally be controlled at a time without interference. Controlled processes are thus tightly capacity-limited, and require more time for their activation. But controlled processes have the advantage of being relatively easy to set up, alter, and apply to novel situations. In this framework, learning involves the transfer of information to long-term memory and is regulated by controlled processes. That is, skills are learned and become automatic only after the earlier use of controlled processes. These are controlled processes that regulate the flow of information from short-term to long-term memory. Individual memory aptitude can be transformed or improved to make language input a permanent state in our memory. Long-term memory seems to offer fairly permanent and unlimited storage capacity for everything that we hold long enough in short-term memory to be processed, understood and deemed worth remembering. Short-term memory is ephemeral and of limited capacity; it can hold about seven chunks of information for a few seconds. A person can retain the contents in short-term memory by repeating them continuously, but once a person stops doing that, they will be lost from short-term memory forever; since short-term memory is ephemeral, once people complete the relevant task, they will almost certainly not remember the details of the information they were using unless something has caused it to be transferred to long-term memory. Learning involves time, but once automatic processes are set up at one stage in the development of a complex information-processing skill, controlled processes are free to be allocated to higher levels of processing. Thus controlled processing can be said to lay down the "stepping stones" for automatic processing as a learner moves to more and more difficult levels (Rodgers, 2007).

There is some evidence (Sachs, 1967) to suggest that "semantic" (i.e., meaning) and "grammatical" information are not treated alike in memory. We find the meanings of sentences easier to recall than their exact grammatical shapes. The exact grammatical form of a sentence is quickly forgotten but the information it contains is not. People remember the substance of what was said much better than they remember how exactly it was conveyed.

It is also scientifically proven that memory has "a beginning effect" and "a final effect". "The beginning effect" of memorising appears just after the beginning of learning; "the final effect" is associated with the end of learning. These effects are closely dependent on "brother-effects" like "the effect of distinction" that stands for creative or even bizarre notions and "the effect of repetitions" that contains multiple need for revisions (Stevick, 1976).

The layers of memory attributes are closely related to the features of memory that any language teacher who motivates learners should be aware of. These are the features of memory that work in correlation (Stevick, 1976):

- the speed of remembering – the number of repetitions needed to consolidate the vocabulary or a structure trace,
- the extent – the number of memorised traces after just one conception,
- fidelity – the consistency (compatibility) with memorising of recorded traces,

- ➢ permanence – the time of keeping traces in memory,
- ➢ readiness – the ease and speed (pace) of recalling.

In the absence of vision, the world is experienced as a sequence of events. Since the visually impaired constantly use serial memory strategies in everyday circumstances, they tend to develop superior skills (Baddeley, 1983).

2.8. The author's three-layer intelligence structure versus Gardner's two-layer intelligence structure

The concept of intelligence encompasses a broad spectrum of abilities, including "verbal fluency, logical ability, and wide general knowledge but common sense, wit, creativity, lack of bias, sensitivity to one's limitations, intellectual independence, openness to experience, and the like" (Neisser, 1979:186).

The involvement of intelligence or multiple intelligences in the process of teaching-learning English as a foreign language to visually impaired students (or any students) is evident to me.

Considering the teaching-learning process, the notion of Gardner's theory of multiple intelligences cannot be omitted. It debunked traditional intelligence testing as inadequate and proposed an alternative way of looking at human intelligence as a plurality of intelligences that develop at different rates and stem from various neurological patterns. Gardner (1993) identifies seven intelligences: logical, visual/spatial, kinaesthetic, linguistic, musical, interpersonal, intrapersonal. By pluralising intelligences in this way he opens the definition of "smart" to allow its application to a variety of gifts, skills and talents. Instead of asking *"Am I smart?"*, the question becomes *"How smart am I?"*

This question: "How smart are my visually impaired students?" accompanied my research-experience during the psycho-linguistic therapy "Touching the World".

I strongly agree with Gardner's view (1993:13) on intelligence:

> To my mind, a human intellectual competence must entail a set of skills of problem solving – enabling the individual to resolve genuine problems or difficulties that he or she encounters and, when appropriate, to create an effective product – and must also entail the potential for finding or creating problems – and thereby laying the groundwork for the acquisition of new knowledge.

I strongly disagree with Gardner's (1993) two-path intelligence structure: the core content and the means, called medium (Figure 6A). The core content is the initial recognition of a learning process and the means is the factor or any aid that stimulates development. He called it "two-layer rule of intelligence".

Figure 6A. Gardner's two-layer intelligence structure

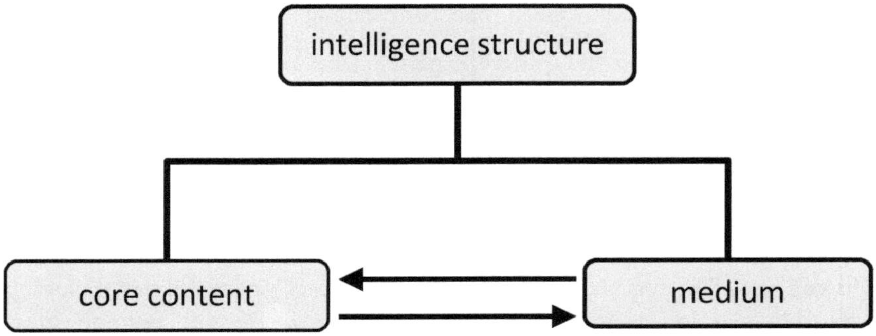

In my view, the structure of intelligence should be analysed as a three-layer intelligence field (Figure 6B) instead of two-layer division; it is worth emphasising that the involvement of intelligence cannot be discussed without the goals = products that stimulate the core content of intelligence and are the basis of any recognition (emphasised in Gardner's definition of intelligence). The core content is flexible and has an influence on its medium layer and the goal content that it meets. The core content and the means are "absorbed" through the process of goal-content achievement. That is why the third layer of intelligence can be seen as an additional value of linguistic-mental involvement of the visually impaired.

I suggest that intelligence itself employs not only one-layer content and the means, called medium, as Gardner emphasised, but the structure is enriched with the support of the additional layer of the content, which appears to be the product of the core content-layer, achieved through the engagement of medium, involved in the process of building intelligence structure. The medium incorporated in the matrix of intelligence correlates with the concept of motivation, its extrinsic and intrinsic layers, and ought to be reconsidered as a sub-means of the medium redevelopment. Gardner suggests that the initial core content equals the final content, not emphasising the key difference between them. The core content is changeable and ought to be recognised on two layered-acquisition – initial and final, understood as the added value, written in the process of creation, reinforced by sensory compensation, unavoidable to be utilised, in the context of the visually impaired process of teaching-learning a foreign language.

Figure 6B. The author's three-layer intelligence structure

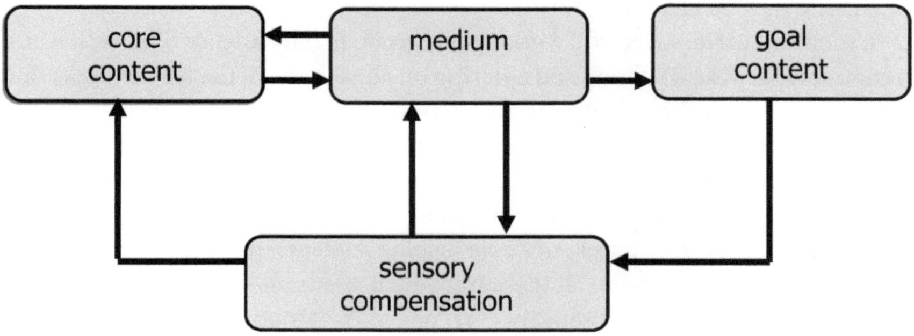

Summing up, the intelligence structure appears to exist as a complex area of consideration-explanation. I found it crucial to enrich Gardner's thesis with the added value – the goal content of the intelligence acquisition involved in the interaction between the core content and medium. The cohesion of the medium with the field of sensory compensation seems to be noticeably reciprocated towards the empowerment of the visually impaired.

2.9. Group therapy space

Freud (1965) said that the goal of therapy was to make the unconscious conscious. The goal of therapy is to provide a nonjudgmental environment. The therapist offers the environment where the person can feel safe in revealing feelings or actions that have led to stress or tension in his/her life. Oftentimes, simply sharing these burdens with other people can have a beneficial influence (Douglas, 1983). Good therapy needs to be more than attention. There is a strong teaching component; teaching, retraining, rethinking, and restructuring need to be included in the change process (Saretsky, 1977).

It is fundamental for success to have support and co-operation from the group and a harmonious relationship between its members. Establishing trust appears to be a crucial link of the group therapy. The group is to be cohesive and work productively if its members know something about each other and are willing to disclose information about themselves. The participants share their feelings and thoughts and give one another feedback, encourage and give support or criticism (McLeish, 1973).

The group can also become a source of strength in times of stress for participants. The feedback a person gets from others can make him/her become aware of maladaptive patterns of behaviour, and help change his/her point of view to adopt more constructive and effective reactions. It can become a laboratory for practising new behaviours.

It is crucial to the successful working of a group to have a sense of direction and a common purpose. Defining and agreeing on aims is one of the hardest tasks that the group has to undertake together. It can be hard for many reasons: students may not have defined their own aims clearly to themselves; they may have only a hazy notion of what therapy involves or they may have very precise and narrow aims of their own, which may conflict with others' aims or the wider aims of the group. The teacher has a difficult task, not only helping students individually clarify their aims, but somehow weaving all these individual wants and needs together into a coherent programme which satisfies everyone in the group. According to the rule "ten pupils ten puppets" (Douglas, 1983), the teacher-therapist ought to imagine that he/she has ten puppets-students, and each one is attached to one of his/her fingers. The teacher manipulates them all separately but gets them to work as a whole.

The PLT was a reeducative group therapy (Wolberg, 1967), focused on achievements in L2 and increasing the intensity of positive affects, leading to modifying behaviour, altering problematic goals, and achieving creative potentialities.

Chapter Three: Linguistic aspects of therapy

3.0. Introductory remarks

Chapter two describes the linguistic aspects of the psycho-linguistic therapy "Touching the World", based on theory of language and theories of language learning: Steven Krashen's Monitor Model, Spolsky, or Mackney. The key method – the Direct Method – was transformed due to its lack of effectiveness and creativity into the Re-charged Direct Method. The support of the Audiolingual Method and Total Physical Response I found crucial to be introduced.

3.1. Language as a means of expressing emotions

Language is possibly the highest mental process or set of processes of all. Language is a system that allows its users to interact with one another; the system that not only allows individual "minds" to function, but also provides a means for sharing the results of that functioning with others (Wardhaugh, 1994). Chomsky (1968) defined language by means of generative grammar: a finite set of rules which would enable users to make an unlimited number of expressions.

Any attempt, therefore, to discuss how language functions in communication requires making a clear distinction between language forms and language functions. Language forms are the phonological, syntactic and semantic properties of language; language functions are the uses speakers make of language forms in communication, i.e., the pragmatic uses of language (Leech, 1990).

A basic assumption behind any attempt to understand language functioning is that most utterances have a purpose – they are spoken with an "intent" to express something (e.g., emotions). The speaker's intention, therefore, is part of the meaning of any utterance.

According to Jakobson (Leech, 1990), language serves the following functions:

- cognitive or referential, to convey messages and information,
- conative, to persuade and influence others through commands and entreaties,
- emotive, to express attitudes, feelings and emotions,
- phatic, to establish communion with others,
- metalingual, to clear up difficulties about intentions, words and meanings,
- poetic, to indulge in language for its own sake.

Another classification, proposed by Halliday (Wardhaugh, 1994), refers to seven different categories of language function: instrumental, regulatory, representational, interactional, personal, heuristic and imaginative. The personal function refers to language used to express the individual's personality. Each individual is conscious of the fact that language comprises part of that individuality. Individuals have a voice in what happens to them. They are also free to speak or not to speak, to say much or as little as they please, and to choose how to say or what they say. Language provides the individual with a means to express emotions, whether outright in the form of exclamations, endorsements or curses, or much more subtly through a careful choice of words. The personal function undoubtedly exists, but it is possibly the most difficult of all functions to describe with any exactness. In that function, language, thoughts, and emotions come together to interact in ways that are still quite mysterious to us.

The following features of language cover the area of emotional expressing (Wardhaugh, 1994):

- Duality of patterns is generally acknowledged to be the most distinctive feature of language. Every human language makes use of two largely independent subsystems, one of sounds and the other of meanings. This feature enables a small number of elements of one subsystem to be combined and recombined into units and patterns of meaning in the other subsystem.
- Semanticity refers to the meaning content of the system.
- Productivity – language is infinitely productive in the variations that can occur in what is said.
- Discreteness refers to the fact that the system is made up of elements that are clearly distinguishable from one another.
- Displacement allows people to construct messages about the past, present and future, and also about both real and imaginary worlds.

These design features are obviously not all completely independent of one another. Some could not exist without others.

Emotions are expressed through language on the basis of various factors (Nowakowska-Kempna, 1995):

(1) prosodical – intonation, accent, the length of vowels, tone of voice,
(2) lexical – exclamations, word repetition, expressive words,
(3) word formation – diminutive, augmentative,
(4) syntax – simple, short sentences, elliptical sentences.

In essence, the number of linguistic means depends on an individual's language communicative competences, social and situational aspects.

According to Wardhaugh (1994), emotions are expressed in two ways: directly and indirectly. They are expressed indirectly by changing the tone of voice, through errors in syntax or disruption of speech. Expressing emotions also relates to certain issues that are not mentioned directly, but are actually being talked around. Sometimes a particular word or sentence quickly opens up or even closes down a whole topic or indicates how issues related to the topic are to be resolved or to be unresolved. Often, expressing emotions accompanies ambiguity, uncertainty, and gaps in information. Vagueness rather than precision often prevails and words are understood metaphorically as well as literally. Items may not be sequenced logically or chronologically, some may not be mentioned at all and others never explained.

Emotions can be also expressed on different levels:

- oral and written,
- verbal and nonverbal.

Nonverbal expressions include body tension, hand and body movements, facial expressions, posture, tone of voice, the amount of physical space between people, variations of speech, any kind of touch. All of these are matters to be considered in the communication process.

The expressive function of language also covers backchannel signals. Advice-seeking and trouble-sharing are typical types of discourse where emotional attitudes become the focus of attention. Common *backchannel signals* show that we do not only hear and are listening to the message but are actively engaged in the interaction. If we withhold backchannel signals, the speaker assumes that we are not listening, that we are bored, or that we disagree with the message. Then, *turn-taking signals* – the turns in a conversation – are symmetric. One person or the other does not dominate without permission. There are lexical phrases that must be used to gain permission for a long turn. Turn-taking signals may be very subtle when the speakers know each other. The rhythm of the conversation is quickly set and each person comes in on cue according to that rhythm. One speaker cues the end of a turn by using falling intonation or stretching final vowels (Hatch and Brown, 1995).

In expressing emotions speakers may vary their rates of speech, loudness, speech rhythms, habits of pausing, amount of talking and even their accents in relation to other participants.

One of the keynotes of the linguistic approach to ***semantics*** is that there is no escape from language. The term semantics refers to the study of meaning and the systematic ways those meanings are expressed in language (Hatch and Brown, 1995).

> Semantics as the study of meaning is central to the study of communication; and as communication becomes more and more a crucial factor in social organisation, the need to understand it becomes more and more pressing. Semantics is also at the centre of the study of the human mind-thought processes, cognition, conceptualisation – all these intricately bound up with the way in which we classify and convey our experience of the world through language (Leech, 1990:ix).

"Meaning is what language is all about" (Langacker, quoted in Kopka, 2002: 7). Meaning is not stable but depends on speakers, hearers, and context. Meaning can be spread over seven different ingredients (Leech, 1990):

- conceptual meaning (or cognitive meaning) – logical, cognitive, or denotative content,
- connotative meaning – what is communicated by virtue of what language refers to,
- social meaning – what is communicated through the social circumstances of language use,
- affective meaning – what is communicated through feelings and attitudes of the speaker,
- reflected meaning – what is communicated through association with another sense of the same expression,
- collocative meaning – what is communicated through association with words which tend to occur in the environment of another word,
- thematic meaning – what is communicated by the way in which the message is organised in terms of order and emphasis.

Language reflects personal feelings of the speaker, including his/her attitude to the listener, or his/her attitude to something he/she is talking about at the level of conceptual, connotative and affective meanings. Affective meaning is often explicitly conveyed through conceptual or connotative content of the words used.

Words do not have meanings in isolation. In general, the meaning of a word is related to the meanings of other words in ways that may be simple or complex (Trask, 1995). According to Yule (1996), the meaning of words is analysed in several different ways in order to account for as many aspects of meaning as possible. First of all, words are considered in terms of their semantic features that are basic elements enabling the differentiation of meaning of words. Apart from semantic features of words, semantic roles are also examined; they describe the way in which words are used in sentences and the functions they fulfil. Thus, the entity that performs an action is known as an agent, while the entity involved in an action is called the theme. When an agent uses an entity in order to do something, this entity is called an instrument. However, when a person in a sentence does not perform any action, but only has a perception, or a state of feeling, then the role is described as the experience. Finally, there are roles connected with motion or position of entities. So, the location is where an entity is, the source is the initial position of the entity, the place is where it moves from and the goal is where the entity moves to. Another issue investigated by semantics is the relationship between words. The simplest relationship between words is synonymy versus antonymy. Sometimes the meaning of one word is included in the meaning of another, broader term. Then the relationship between words can be described as hyponymy. Another interesting relation between words is that of metonymy, which is based on a close connection of certain entities in everyday experience. The connection can be that of container-content, whole-part, or others.

Semantics is a veritable element in the study on emotions. In Bloomfield's words (Leech, 1990), the meaning of a word should be studied as part of the human being's emotional and biological make-up. According to Wierzbicka (1971:34), the semantic analysis of emotions can be considered on three layers:

(1) the correlation between emotion and the event-cause,
(2) the correlation between emotion and body-effect,
(3) the correlation between emotion and the event, not necessarily being the effect or the cause of the emotion, but being the effect of the same causes as the emotion.

Words as symbols are effective instruments in the analysis of emotions and reflect their intensity. Wierzbicka (1999:2) claimed that "the meaning of the English word emotion includes both a reference to feeling and a reference to thought (as well as a reference to the body)".

The analysis of the language of emotion (Maia, 1998) is closely related to the lexical point of view. Emotion is a phenomenon that can take different syntactic forms, which may evince greater or lesser rationalisation about the emotion, according to their complexity. "It may be a simple noun, which signifies that the Senser (a person who feels emotion) has only focused on some person or object, … or it may be a complete clause" (Maia, 1998:215). A tendency to favour the noun form is clearly visible when discussing individual items. The verbs of emotions are divided into two classes: dynamic verbs and static verbs. There is a tendency to use have + emotion noun, where the subject has an emotion – rather than being emotional – thus semantically distinguishing between the subject and the emotion. The reflexive *-se* is generally used with psychological verbs. Due to a trace of reflexivity it suggests that the subject plays a role in the emotion process that is actually built into the semantics of the syntax. Maia also emphasises the metaphorical description of emotions – from physically based metaphors to highly culturally based ones.

In essence, emotions in language cannot be expressed or "discovered" without their attributions to meanings and values.

3.2. Theory of language learning: Steven Krashen's Monitor Model

In Diller's words "a living language is characterised by rule-governed creativity" (Mitchell and Myles, 2002:16). This principle is clearly based on two concepts: language is rule-governed and creative. This implies teaching a language as a consciously learnt system.

The language acquisition process is guided by theory. Theory is implicit in the practice of language teaching. It reveals itself in the assumptions underlying practice, in the planning of a course of study, in the routines of the classroom, in value judgments about language teaching, and in the decisions that a language teacher has to make day by day.

Theory development makes language teaching more meaningful and intellectually more satisfying (Stern, 1994:27).

> A theory views a topic or certain practical activities as something coherent and unified, but divisible into parts. A theory offers a system of thought, a method of analysis and synthesis, or a conceptual framework in which to place different observations, phenomena, or activities. It is in this widest sense that we can also speak of theory of second language teaching.

Each theory has a worldview that should be compatible with the attitudes and values of the teacher. Moreover, each theory demands a skill set to be delivered that involves a structure. Finally, the theory used, ought to be effectively enacted.

Under theory, it is possible to subsume different schools of thought, each with their own assumptions, postulates, principles, models, and concepts. These are what are often referred to as language teaching methods, approaches, philosophies, or schools of thought.

In my view, the most ambitious and convincing theory of the second-language learning process is Krashen's Monitor Model. The Monitor Model of second language development is an example of a learning theory on which the Natural Approach was built. The Monitor theory (Krashen, 1985) addresses both the process and the condition dimensions of learning. At the level of the process, Krashen distinguishes between acquisition and learning. Acquisition refers to the natural assimilation of language rules through using language for communication.

Learning refers to the formal study of language rules and is a conscious process. According to Krashen, however, learning is available only as a "monitor". The monitor is the repository of conscious grammatical knowledge about a language that is learned through formal instruction and that is called upon in the editing of utterances produced through the acquired system. Krashen's theory also addresses the conditions necessary for the process of acquisition to take place. He describes these in terms of the type of input the learner receives. Input must be comprehensible, slightly above the learner's present level of competence, interesting or relevant, not grammatically sequenced. His theory is to be placed on the deductive side of the inductive-deductive continuum. That is, the theory begins with a number of assumptions, from which definite hypotheses are derived:

1. *The Acquisition-Learning Hypothesis* – Krashen maintained that adult second language learners have at their disposal two distinct and independent ways of developing competence in a second language: acquisition, which is "a subconscious process identical in all ways to the process children utilise in acquiring their first language" (1985:8) and learning which is "a conscious process that results in knowing about language" (ibidem). Acquisition comes about through meaningful interaction in a natural communication setting. Speakers are not concerned with form, but with meaning; nor is there explicit concern with error detection and correlation. This contrasts with the language learning situation in which error detection and correction are central. It is important to Krashen to make a clear distinction between conscious and unconscious. He does not provide definitions of these terms, although he does operationally identify conscious learning with judgements of grammaticality based on "rule" and subconscious acquisition with judgements based on "feel" (Krashen, 1978). The difficulty with such an approach is that it is impossible to know whether subjects in this experiment were actually operating on the basis of "rule" or "feel".
2. *The Monitor Hypothesis* states that "learning has only one function, and that is a monitor or editor", and that learning comes into play only to "make changes in the form of our utterance, after it has been produced by the acquired system" (Krashen, 1985:15). The Monitor is thought to alter the output of the acquired system before or after utterance is actually written or spoken, but the utterance is initiated entirely by the acquired system. Krashen's position is that conscious knowledge of rules does not help acquisition, but only enables a learner to "polish up" what has been acquired through communication. The focus of language teaching, for him, should not be rule-learning but communication.

3. *The Natural Order Hypothesis* states that learners' progress is seen through "natural" developmental sequences:

> We acquire the rules of language in a predictable order, some rules tending to come early and others late. The order does not appear to be determined solely by formal simplicity and there is evidence that it is independent of the order in which rules are taught in language classes (Krashen, 1985:21).

This "natural" order of acquisition is presumed to be the result of the acquired system, operating free of conscious grammar, or the Monitor.

4. *The Input Hypothesis* is analysed through two corollaries:
   - Speaking is a result of acquisition and not its cause. Speech cannot be taught directly but emerges on its own as a result of building competence via comprehensible input.
   - If input is understood, and there is enough of it, the necessary grammar is automatically provided.

Thus for Krashen, comprehensible input is the route to acquisition and to information about grammar in the target language, and is automatically available when the input is understood.

5. *The Affective Filter Hypothesis* claims that comprehensible input may not be utilised by second-language acquirers if there is a mental block that prevents them from fully profiting from it. The affective filter acts as a barrier to acquisition: if the filter is down, the input reaches the Language Acquisition Device (LAD) and becomes acquired competence; if the filter is up, the input is blocked and does not reach the LAD. This occurs when an acquirer is unmotivated, lacking in confidence, or concerned with failure. For Krashen, the effective filter is the principal source of individual differences in second language acquisition:

> The Affective Filter Hypothesis captures the relationship between affective variables and the process of second language acquisition by positing that acquirers vary with respect to the strength or level of their affective filters. Those whose attitudes are not optimal for second language acquisition will not only tend to seek less input, but they will also have a high or strong affective filter – even if they understand the message, the input will not reach that part of the brain responsible for language acquisition, or the LAD. Those with attitudes more conducive to second language acquisition will not only seek and obtain more input, they will also have a lower or weaker filter (1985:31).

The filter is described as having four functions:

- It determines which language models a learner will select.
- It determines which part of the language will be attended to first.

- It determines when the language acquisition efforts should cease.
- It determines how fast a learner can acquire a language.

Thus the argument is that a strong or high affective filter blocks input from reaching the LAD. The filter is thought to limit what will be learnt, and how quickly the language will be acquired.

The affective filter was first proposed by Dulay and Burt (1982: 46) to account for how affective variables affect the process of second-language learning. In their work the affective filter was defined as follows: "The filter is that part of the internal processing system that subconsciously screens incoming language based on what psychologists call *affect*: the learner's motives, needs, attitudes, and emotional states".

In essence, language teaching-learning theory has been in contact with psychology; psychology directs attention to the individual person as a language user and as a language learner. Since language teaching is concerned with the acquisition by individuals of a dual language command, its theory is bound to operate with psychological concepts of language use and language learning, and psychological thinking on these topics forms an essential part of any language teaching theory.

3.3. Theoretical framework on language teaching models

I found three models of language teaching essential to be analysed in my thesis:

- Spolsky's educational linguistics model,
- Mackey's interaction model,
- Stern's four-component model.

According to Spolsky (1989), the model of language teaching has three main sources:

1. language description,
2. a theory of language learning,
3. a theory of language use.

A theory of language learning must ultimately derive from a theory of language and a theory of learning. Language description must also be founded in a theory of language. The disciplines that provide the necessary theoretical foundations and the data underlying language teaching are psychology for the theory of learning, psycholinguistics for the theory of language learning, and general linguistics for a theory of language and language descriptions. These disciplines come together in dealing with the problem of language education and thus constitute a problem-oriented discipline which Spolsky calls educational linguistics – applied linguistics. What Spolsky's model makes particularly clear are the main components of a language teaching theory, and the specific role that each discipline performs in relation to these components.

Mackey (Mitchell and Myles, 2002:89) identifies five major variables in his interaction model:

- **M** – methods and materials,
- **T** – what a teacher does,
- **I** – instruction: what a learner gets,
- **S** – sociolinguistic and sociocultural influences of the environment,
- **L** – what a learner does.

Mackey's conceptual framework indicates how the teaching variables (MTI) as well as the learning variables (ISL) are dependent upon social and educational factors. Mackey describes the model of interdisciplinary framework involving such sciences as psychology, sociology, anthropology, education and linguistics.

Stern (1994) depicts the model of language teaching that is operated with four key concepts: language, learning, teaching and context. Language teaching requires a concept of the nature of language. Implicitly, the teacher works with a theory of language. Language teaching demands a view of the learner and the nature of language learning. The fundamental questions are: *What language learner does this theory envisage?* And, *How does it view language learning?* The disciplines which most directly relate to this question are psychology, particularly educational psychology, and psycholinguistics for language learning and language use. Language teaching implies a view of the language teacher and language teaching. Finally, language teaching occurs in a given context. The interpretation of the context is an essential part of theory.

These various models have a great deal in common. They suggest that there is a consensus about factors and issues that should be taken into account in developing a language teaching theory. They also recognise the interaction of a multiplicity of factors; they are interdisciplinary.

3.4. Approach, method, and technique

At least three different views of language and the nature of language proficiency explicitly or implicitly inform current approaches and methods in language teaching (Richards and Rodgers, 2001).

The first and the most traditional of the three is the structural view that is related to language as a system of structurally related elements for the coding of meaning. The target of language learning is seen to be the mastery of elements of this system: grammatical units, grammatical operations and lexical items. The Audiolingual Method embodies this particular view of language, as do such contemporary methods as Total Physical Response.

The second view of language is the functional view – language is a vehicle for the expression of functional meaning. The communicative movement in language teaching subscribes to this view of language. This theory emphasises the semantic and communicative dimension rather than merely the grammatical characteristics of language, and leads to a specification and organisation of language teaching content by categories of meaning and function rather than by elements of structure and grammar, just as the Direct Method emphasises.

The third view of language can be called the interactional view. It sees language as a vehicle for the realisation of interpersonal relations and for the performance of social transactions between individuals. Language is seen as a tool for creation and maintenance of social relations. Interactional theories focus on the patterns of moves, acts, negotiations, and interactions found in conversational exchanges. Language teaching content, according to this view, may be specified and organised by patterns of exchange and interaction or may be left unspecified, to be shaped by the inclinations of learners or interactors. The Direct Method issues incline towards this view.

In 1963, Anthony formulated a framework to describe foreign language teaching and learning within three levels: approach, method and technique (Anthony, quoted in Richards and Rogers, 2001:19).

> An *approach* is a set of correlative assumptions dealing with the nature of language teaching and learning; it describes the nature of the subject matter to be taught; it is axiomatic (clear, does not need to be proved). A *method* is an overall plan for the orderly presentation of language material, no part of which contradicts, and all of which is based upon the selected approach; a method is procedural. Within one approach, there can be methods. A *technique* is implementational – that which actually takes place in a classroom. It is a particular trick, stratagem or contrivance used to accomplish an immediate objective. Technique must be consistent with a method and therefore in harmony with an approach.

According to Anthony, "the arrangement is hierarchical; the organizational key is that techniques carry out a method which is consistent with an approach..." (Anthony, quoted in Richards and Rogers, 2001:19). Anthony's model presents *approach*, which is the level at which assumptions and beliefs about language and language learning are specified; *method*, which is the level at which theory is put into practice and at which choices are made about particular skills, the content to be taught, and the order in which the content will be presented; and *technique*, which is related to the level at which classroom procedures are described (Anthony, 1963). Anthony's framework is seen as a useful way of classifying different teaching practices. However, it does not clearly define the difference between approach, method, and technique. Kumaravadivelu (2006:85) reports that due to this ambiguity there was "widespread dissatisfaction" with it. Anthony himself recognised the limitations of his framework, and was open to the idea of improvements being made to it.

Richards and Rogers' 1982 approach was expanded on Anthony's three-level framework; instead of approach, method, and technique, they chose the terms: approach, design, and procedure. Their concept of approach was similar to Anthony's, but their design and procedure were of a broader scope than Anthony's method and technique. Their design referred to all major practical implications in the classroom, such as syllabus design, types of activities to be used in the classroom, students' and teachers' roles; procedure referred to different behaviours, practices and techniques observed in the classroom. These new terms were intended to address limitations in Anthony's purely descriptive framework and also gave them specific criteria by which they could evaluate different methods. Their framework has been criticised by Kurmaravadielu for having "an element of artificiality in its conception and an element of subjectivity in its operation" (2006:87).

Lewis (1993:15) states that "an approach is an integrated set of theoretical and practical beliefs, embodying syllabus and method. If syllabus is the what of language teaching, and method the how, approach is the why"; he considers the rule of "what-how-why" as a clearly understood key to teaching-learning a foreign language.

It should be emphasised that "important differences between teaching normally sighted and visually impaired students occur at the level of techniques" (Krzeszowski, 2012: 40). The involvement of visual impairment in the process of teaching and learning a foreign language causes modifications at the level of techniques, related to didactic aids, based on sensory compensation and time spent on performing certain tasks (Figure 7).

In essence, "approach is defined a priori, which means that its claims are based on theoretical considerations and can be verified in practice at the level of techniques" (Krzeszowski, 2012:39).

Figure 7. The author's circular model of approach, method, and technique related to visual impairment

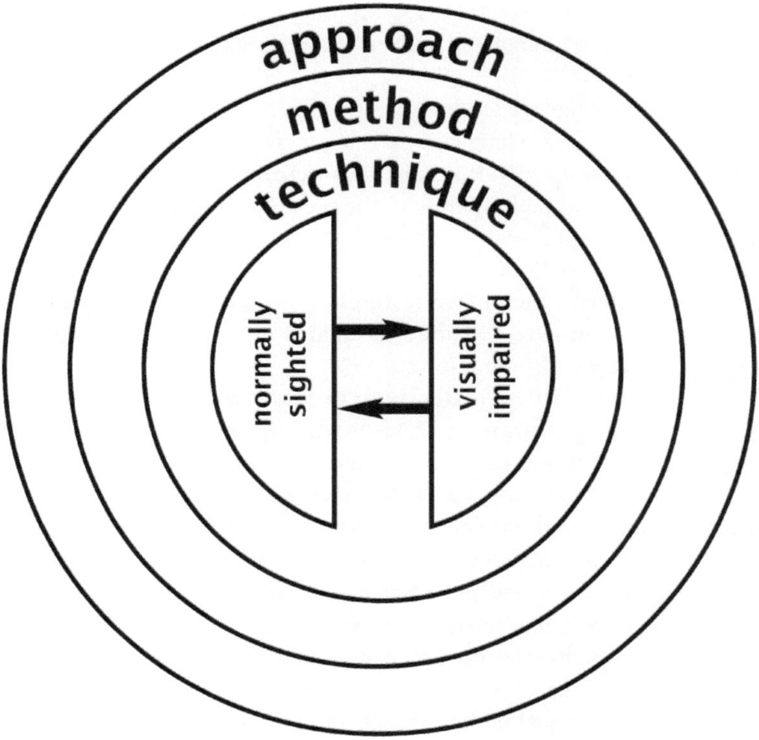

In my thesis, I found three methods crucial within language learning theory: the main one – the Direct Method, and supportive ones – the Audiolingual Method and Total Physical Response.

These will be depicted in the next subchapters.

3.5. Direct Method issues

The main question guiding this study was concerned with the linguistic theory basis that provides an adequate language relation to visually impaired students. The choice to embody the Direct Method in the PLT process was not accidental. Because of my teaching experience I was engrossed in the main guidance of this method that aims at the effectively achieved communicative approach and question-answer interaction between a teacher and a student. The aspect of repetitions and the frequency of teacher-student correlations have become the perceptible modules of the methodological usage. The sensory compensation issue was the priority to be analysed in the method formation for the students with visual disorders.

Historically, the language teaching reforms from 1850 to 1900, particularly in Europe, attempted to make language teaching more effective by a radical change from grammar-translation. Various methods were developed during this period attesting to the general discontent with the prevailing theory and practice. The proposed reforms went under a variety of names: the Reform Method, Natural Method, Phonetical Method or Anti-grammatical Method, but the most persistent term to describe the various features of the new approaches in language teaching was the term Direct Method, as an answer to the shortcomings of the Grammar Translation Method (Howatt, 1984).

The impetus to the Direct Method can be partly attributed to practical unconventional teaching reformers who responded to the need for better language learning in a new world of industry and international trade and travel such as Berlitz and Gouin. It was partly also stimulated by linguistic scholarship, linguistic theory, philology, and phonetics. The development of the Direct Method is closely linked with the introduction of phonetics into language pedagogy. Both phonetics and the Direct Method emphasised the use of the spoken language. Conceptually, however, they are not necessarily linked.

The lack of comprehensive documentation of this important development in language pedagogy is an obstacle to in-depth analysis. Kelly is the most accessible source for a historical interpretation, although his treatment of the Direct Method is scattered over different chapters of his work. A systematic attempt to trace the origins and development of the Direct Method in Germany was made by Rulcker (Richards and Rogers, 1991).

The Direct Method psychology is avowedly behaviouristic. Mainly following Skinner, but also influenced by neobehaviourists such as Osgood, its psychology is an interpretation of language learning in terms of stimulus and response, operant conditioning, and reinforcement with an emphasis on successful error-free learning in small well-prepared steps (Carroll, 1966).

The method operates on the idea that second language acquisition ought to be an imitation of first language learning (Rodgers, 2001). Charles Berlitz's method focuses on comparison and similarity findings between first and second language acquisition. In this light, the method employed a lot of oral interaction, spontaneous use of language, and no translation was provided. The method relies on a step-by-step progression based on question-answer sessions. The reason for using questions that require first a negative answer is to force the student to recall the word which is opposite in meaning to the one in the question. The usage of long sentences forces students to speak as much as possible – more than the teacher in fact, which is always desirable. In this way, the student also gets ample opportunity to practice pronunciation. Since the Direct Method class involves much use of the spoken language, stress is also laid on the acquisition of good pronunciation.

The principles of the Direct Method (Howatt, 1984):

- Both speech and listening comprehension are taught.
- Students are taught from the start to ask questions as well as answer them.
- Oral communication skills are built in a carefully graded progression organised around question-answer exchanges between teachers and students in small, intensive groups, supported by regular revisions.
- New teaching points are introduced orally.
- Concrete vocabulary is taught through demonstrations, objects and pictures; abstract vocabulary is taught by association of ideas.
- Only everyday vocabulary and sentences are taught during the initial phase; grammar, reading and writing are introduced in the intermediate phase.
- Grammar is taught inductively.
- The student should be speaking at least 80% of the time during the lesson.
- The emphasis is put on the error correction aspect, aiming at the development of correct pronunciation.
- Classroom instructions are conducted exclusively in the target language.

Some major problems have persistently troubled the Direct Method teaching: how to convey meaning without translating, how to safeguard against misunderstanding without reference to the first language, and finally, how to apply the Direct Method beyond elementary stages (because it was addressed to elementary language competences). The Direct Method extended the repertoire of language instruction in the early stages of teaching, but added relatively little to the teaching of advanced learners.

Summing up, the Direct Method was the first of the methods in which the impetus came both from the inventiveness of a few practitioners and from the critical and theoretical thinking about the nature of language and language learning of a few linguistic scholars such as Sweet and Vietor. The use of a text as a basis of language learning, demonstrations of pictures and objects, the emphasis on question-answer work, spoken narratives, and dictations resulted from the Direct Method. On the L1-L2 issue, the method constitutes a radical attempt to exclude L1 in L2.

3.6. The Audiolingual Method

The Audiolingual Method was involved in the linguistic basis of the PLT. The method supported the Re-charged Direct Method.

The origins of audiolingualism are to be found in the "Army Method" of American wartime language programmes during World War II. A distinct audiolingual method can hardly be identified until the late fifties. It appeared under various names. In the fifties it was most frequently referred to as the aural-oral method. The term "audiolingual" was proposed by Brooks as a more pronounceable alternative (Rodgers, 2001). Brooks also popularised another term, which referred to the same method as "New Key", a term derived from the work by Langer, *Philosophy in a New Key*. Carroll (1966) called the method the "audiolingual habit theory", while the *Pennsylvania Study* referred to it as the "functional skills strategy". Whatever it was called, its period of clearest definition as a distinct language teaching theory and of greatest influence was quite brief; it lasted from about 1959 to 1966. From the beginning of this period, but increasingly so after 1964, audiolingualism has been challenged.

The following principal features of the method (Richards and Rogers, 1991) correspond with the PLT:

- Separation of the skills – listening, speaking, reading, and writing – and the primacy of the audiolingual over the graphic skills: the dominant emphasis is placed on "the fundamental skills" – listening and speaking. Reading and writing are not neglected, but listening and speaking are given priority. Like the Direct Method, audiolingualism tried to develop target skills without reference to the mother tongue. Language learning, in the first instance, was viewed as the acquisition of a practical set of communicative skills; speaking was brought right into the centre of the stage.
- The use of dialogues as the chief means of presenting the language.
- The use of the first language in the language class or in learning materials is not as severely restricted in the Audiolingual Method as it was in the Direct Method.
- It favours an implicit rather than an explicit learning strategy. An emphasis is laid on active and simple practice. The intention is to make language learning more a matter of relatively effortless and frequent repetition and imitation; focus is on memorisation of dialogues and imitative repetition (mimicry) as specific learning techniques.
- The simplicity and directness of approach that was advocated seemed to bring language learning within the scope of the ordinary learner.

- Establishing a linguistic and psychological theory as a basis for the teaching method. The audiolingual theory was probably the first language teaching theory that openly claimed to be derived from linguistics and psychology.

The early development of its linguistic principles was traced by Moulton (Richards and Rogers, 1991). Detailed analytical and critical studies, from a present-day perspective, of the origins, development and impact of audiolingualism are lacking.

3.7. Total Physical Response

Total Physical Response was implemented in the PLT, especially in its linguistic aspect, supporting "vocabulary movement – word segmentation" (discussed in subchapter 5.6.2); and being rooted in the edu-kinaesthetic area (described in subchapter 4.5).

TPR is a language learning method based on the coordination of speech and action. It was developed by James Asher in the 1970s (Krashen and Terrell, 1983). The method uses physical movement to react to verbal input in order to reduce students' inhibitions, lower their effective filter and, in my view, make the visually impaired feel kinaesthetically free, within verbal-physical involvement. TPR facilitates long-term retention of language items and constant repetitions, reducing students' anxiety and stress. It is closely linked to the trace theory of memory, which holds that the more often or intensively a memory connection is traced, the more stronger the memory acts (Stevick, 1976).

Asher emphasised TPR principles, ones he himself elaborated, that seemed to be similar to those brought forward by behavioural psychologists (Rodgers, 2001):

- when language is taught actively through movement, the right hemisphere "believes" and retains it;
- second language learning is parallel to first language learning and should reflect the same naturalistic processes;
- listening should be developed before speaking;
- once listening comprehension has been developed, speech develops naturally and effortlessly out of it;
- delaying speech reduces stress (listening first acquired).

TPR requires instant reactions; students can break the habit of over-analysing language and become more comfortable with "going with the flow", or guessing from the context.

In order to implement TPR effectively, it was necessary to plan regular sessions during the "Touching the World" therapy that progress in a logical, well-organised way.

Chapter Four: The psycho-linguistic therapy "Touching the World" – the experimental method of language teaching for visually impaired students

4.0. Introductory remarks

The main question guiding this chapter is concerned with the consideration of the psycho-linguistic therapy "Touching the World" within two-layered recognition. The mental layer affects the psyche through sandtray therapy, controlled breathing practice, the Brain Linkage Method, and the edu-kinaesthetic area. The linguistic layer offers a two-path differentiation. The lexical and grammar aspects have been analysed through the Re-charged Direct Method, supported with collage and water clusters, involving the media of sand and water, and definite techniques within the area of tactile-audible perception.

4.1. The psycho-linguistic therapy "Touching the World" structure

I designed the psycho-linguistic therapy "Touching the World" to help visually impaired students achieve language competences, developed in parallel, with the process of overcoming mental blockers. The PLT embodies two layers of achievement – linguistic and mental (Figure 8).

Figure 8. The PLT typology area

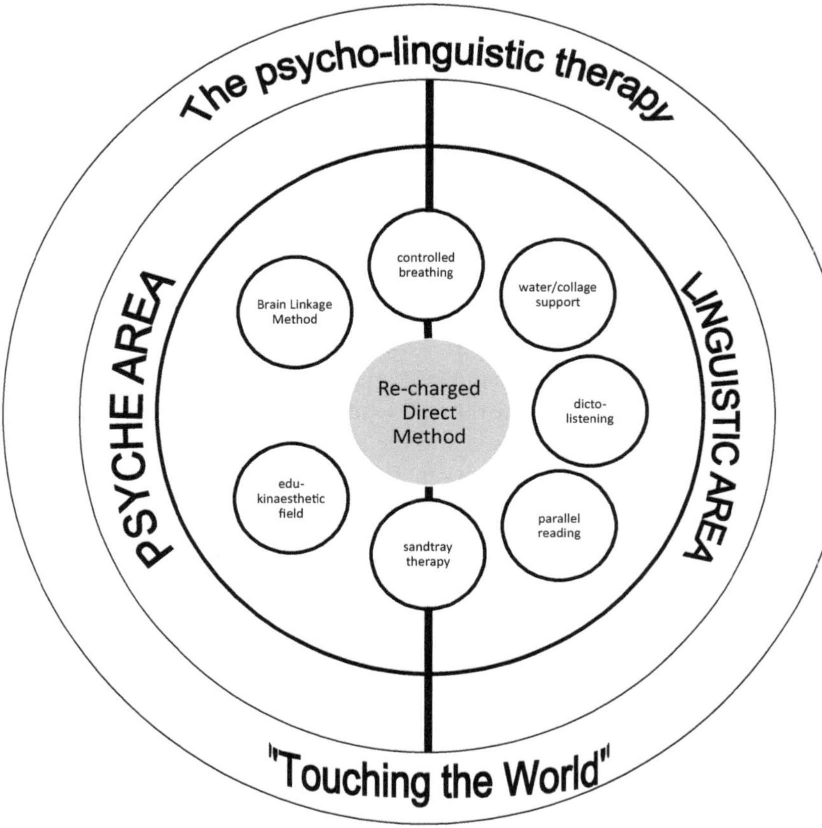

The linguistic layer was acquired through the Re-charged Direct Method based on the Direct Method issues, focused on question-answer interactions and enriched with two supports. Collage support is related to vocabulary teaching, whereas water support covers the field of grammar. Vocabulary development is achieved through word segmentation tasks which focus on the syllable division of each learnt-taught word to reinforce the process of memorising. The grammar area is built through tactile repetition structures, associated with the involvement of haptic perception, practised within definite techniques: ping-pong sentence structure, tactile knots, and the magnetic sentence system (subchapter 5.7). The usage of tactile repetition structures enables students to become hapticly empowered in the process of effective grammar modules building, while simultaneously involved in speaking comprehension (Figure 9).

Figure 9. The PLT linguistic layered recognition

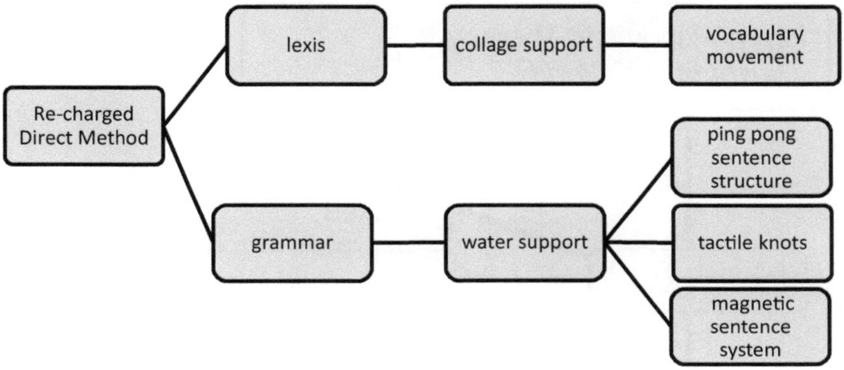

This clear division between lexis and grammar brings students close to efficient recognition of structures, parts of speech, and the order of their appearance. The Re-charged Direct Method also consolidates the clusters of parallel reading and dicto-listening within a speaking skill (subchapter 4.2.2.).

The mental field pivots on emotional openness and mental balance, gained through core issues: the sandtray therapy that covers not only mental but also the linguistic layer of engagement. The controlled breathing area (subchapter 4.2.1.) that focuses on breathing techniques practice, has a supportive role on the mental, but at the same time, the linguistic layer. Then, bioemanation (subchapter 4.4.) correlating with the radiation of hemispheres leads to mental balance development, concentration and memory improvement. The edu-kinaesthetic area (subchapter 4.5.) was also taken into consideration on the basis of the "brain gym" that employs the kinaesthetic aspect of mental support.

The PLT structure (Figure 10) incorporates segmental areas starting from *feedbacks* (Relaxed, Re-charged Water and Re-charged Collage) through *clusters* (Re-charged Direct Method, Controlled Breathing, Edu-Kinaesthetic Area, the Brain Linkage Method, Collage Support, Water Support, and Discussion Zone), then *chains* with the involvement of thematic areas, and finally, *tasks*, focused on definite activities. Each segment grows into definite issues of involvement. Each feedback implies definite clusters. Each cluster incorporates certain chains. In each context chain, diverse tasks are included. The noticeable connection between the sequence of definite clusters and the time schedule leads to achieving a mentally safe zone through learnt-taught language.

Figure 10. The PLT structure

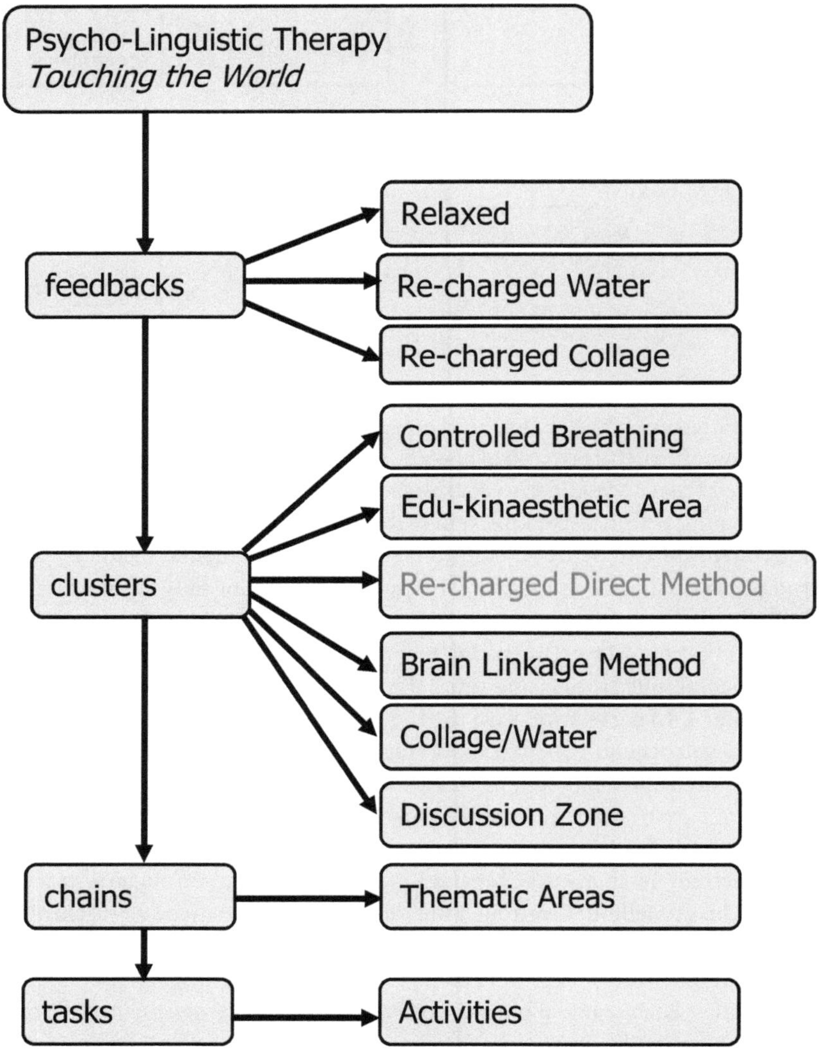

All clusters will be presented in the following subchapters.

4.2. The Re-charged Direct Method

The Re-charged Direct Method cluster, as the name itself indicates, is based on the Direct Method question-answer interaction. The modified, re-charged version comprises three modules: 4-second acquisition (covered in subchapter 4.2.1.), speaking comprehension, and parallel reading or dicto-listening (depicted in subchapter 4.2.2.).

The Re-charged Direct Method operates on the "*3-P rule*" (Harmer, 2004); 4-second acquisition works as the *presentation* of new structures, then speaking comprehension focuses on *practising* them, and finally *production* (in the author's view, production means practice), achieved through parallel reading and dicto-listening. Multiple revisions through the "*3-P rule*" emphasise the adequate rate of the acquisition of lexical and grammar structures.

The procedures of the Direct Method implemented in the Re-charged Direct Method (Krause, 1916):

1. Introduction of a new word, sentence or concept (referred to as an "element") is presented through:
   - Showing – pointing to a visual aid, ensuring that a student clearly understands what is being taught (visually impaired students – tactile graphics involvement).
   - Saying – a teacher verbally introduces an "element", with care and enunciation.
   - Trying – a student makes various attempts to pronounce the new "element".
   - Moulding – a teacher corrects a student if necessary, pointing to show the proper shaping of lips, tongue, and the relationship to the teeth.
   - Repeating – a student repeats each "element" 5–20 times.
2. Syntax, the correct location of the new "element" in the sentence is introduced by:
   - Saying and repeating – a teacher states a phrase or sentence to a student; a student repeats it 5–20 times.
   - Asking and replying in negative – a teacher uses an "element" in negative situations, a student says '*No*'.
   - Interrogatives – a teacher provides intuitive examples using the five-W's (who, what, where, why, when) or how.
3. Progress from one new "element" to another new "element" could be analysed by random sequencing:
   - after the new "element" (X) is taught and learned, going to the next "element" (Y),

- after the next "element" (Y) is taught and learned, returning to practise with the previous "element" (X),
- after these two are alternated (X-Y, Y-X), then going to the third (Z),
- going back to 1 and 2, mixing in three, practising (X-Y-Z, Z-Y-X, Y-Y-Z) and continuing building up to an appropriate number of "elements" (as many as 20 may appear per lesson).

4. Progress from lesson to lesson is reconsidered through:
   1) a lesson review – the first few minutes of each lesson are to review prior lessons.
   2) a global review – the transition from a lesson review to a comprehensive review, which should always include items from the thematic list.

The practical implication is presented in the empirical part (subchapter 5.2).

4.2.1. Controlled breathing

The controlled breathing cluster is a support for the Re-charged Direct Method. It focuses on relaxation techniques that organise learners' abilities to breathe in a certain way, called "the rule of the triple breath", that leads to linguistic development through the auditory channel practice.

Diaphragmatic breathing or belly breathing is an efficient way to release mental and physical stress and tension. It calms the mind and induces a state of relaxation. Students are taught to isolate three areas: the head, chest and abdomen. They can really feel the breath moving through the parts of their bodies (Sisson, 2009). Students inhale deeply, then they exhale imagining that all the stress, tension, and anxiety are being released from their bodies.

During the research the breath itself was first observed, then the awareness of it leading to controlled breathing practice, within 30/2 beats per minute (Figure 11).

Figure 11. Breathing chain – the triple breath rule

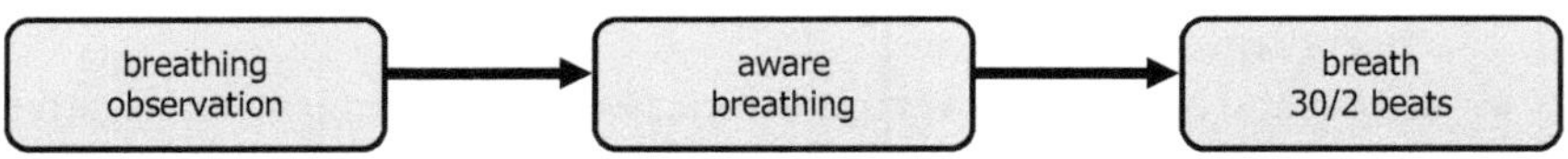

The controlled breathing cluster consists of two segments: **pre-controlled breathing** that leads to **controlled breathing**.

- **Pre-controlled breathing** appears during four sessions of the Relaxed Feedback. It was formed to teach students proper breathing procedures; it is the introduction to controlled breathing. It consists of 10-minute *metronome* *listening* that helps students observe breath itself as a segment factor of this therapy. The metronome sounds at 60–64 beats per minute. The process of breathing starts at three-stage metronome beating: 40/2 beats, 35/2 beats, 30/2 beats – it is advisable to focus on 2 beats, not 30/3 beats, because the inhalation process is transferred into holding a breath, hence 1 beat on inhalation is spread and the second one is spent on exhalation. The students listen to the metronome beating, then count to 4. Afterwards they count and breathe simultaneously, in the rhythm of counting. This element is defined as *breath counting*, covering the cycle of four-second inhalation, then four-second holding of a breath, and four-second exhalation; it takes 5 minutes.

- **Controlled breathing** was created for the Re-charged Direct Method cluster to present new question-answer interaction within the process of 4-second acquisition. The cluster is divided into three cycles (Figure 12):
  (1) the empty cycle (only breathing and counting to 4),
  (2) the primary cycle (the first presentation of new material),
  (3) the secondary cycle (the second presentation of the newly taught material).

In essence, 3 cycles of breath form a circle that cooperate within the 48-second process of 4-second acquisition, which means that one circle equals one structure.

Figure 12. The circle of 4-second acquisition process

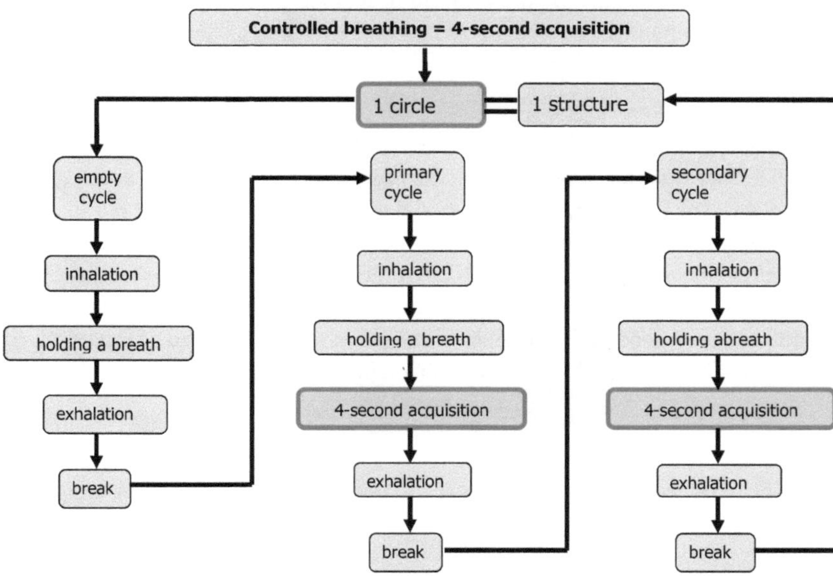

During the 4-second holding of a breath phase, in primary and secondary cycles, the teacher reads new material – 10 structures – while students listen to them, without oral repetitions. One question/answer (based on the issues given during speaking comprehension of the Re-charged Direct question-answer tasks) is introduced twice in the 4-second primary cycle, then repeated twice again in the secondary cycle; one cycle covers three phases, and a break that equals 16 seconds.

Controlled breathing has just one shared field with the suggestopedic issue: material is presented during the holding of a breath phase; the suggestopedia pattern covers 2-second inhalation, 4-second holding of a breath, and 2-second exhalation (Lozanov, 1978). During my research I found the 4s-4s-4s model more efficient in the process of L2 acquisition.

The practical implication is presented in the empirical part (subchapter 5.2).

4.2.2. Supportive issues: parallel reading and dicto-listening

The Re-charged Direct Method has been intentionally extended to parallel reading and dicto-listening. The modifications of typical reading and listening to parallel reading, involving mechanically followed speaking skills, and dicto-listening, emphasise a noticeable skills transfer from receptive (listening, reading) to productive ones (parallel reading and dicto-listening act in a reciprocal arrangement with speaking involvement).

Parallel reading

It is obvious that the blind cannot do the readings (other than in Braille, if they know it). That was the reason for the creation of parallel reading, working in a definite way: the teacher reads the material that has been prepared before, and a student is one word behind the teacher. The blind or visually impaired students repeat after the teacher separate words that are joined in one structure; they do not make mistakes because they follow the teacher's pronunciation. It sounds as an audible one-voiced path; students are heard in the foreground of the teacher's voice, which is distinctly located in the background (Figure 13).

Figure 13. Parallel reading

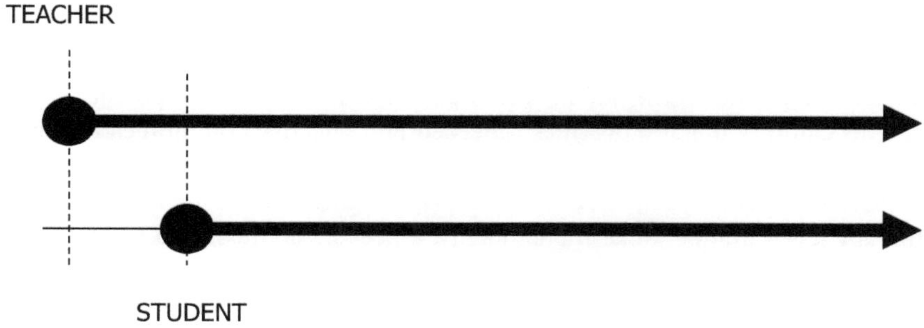

Dicto-listening

The students with visual disorders cannot write dictations (except in Braille, if they know it). This was the reason for changing a dictation into a dicto-gloss, which was a core to creating dicto-listening. A dicto-gloss is a task-based procedure designed to help language-learning students towards a better understanding of how grammar works on a text basis (Llewelyn, 1989). The resemblance of a dicto-gloss and traditional dictation is only superficial (Davis and Rinvolucri, 1987). The analogy begins and ends with the fact that in both a passage is dictated. In a dicto-gloss, the style of dictating, the focus on a text approach to grammar, the task that follows are all totally different. Here, the learners are obliged to create their own parallel texts (Hannan, 1989).

A dicto-listening is a short text in the PLT process based upon a question-answer text (the revision of the structures, introduced during the 4-second acquisition process, then practised during speaking comprehension) that is read twice or three times, at normal speed, to a class of learners who jot down familiar words or phrases in their minds, in the order of their appearance, and/or choose objects, miniatures or realia to design sandtrays (individually or in pairs). Then the students pool their texts and strive to reconstruct their version of the original text from their shared-mind resources. Each group of students produces its own reconstructed version, aiming at grammatical accuracy and textual cohesion, but not at replicating the original text. Diverse versions are analysed and compared, then the students refine their own texts in the light of the shared scrutiny and discussion.

In essence, parallel reading and dicto-listening offer reinforcement of reading and listening skills, especially directed to the linguistic education of the visually impaired.

4.3. The sandtray therapy

The PLT involves the procedure that is called the sandtray therapy. It works as a double tool: on the one hand a mentally effective aid, correlated with a positive affects change and on the other a didactic means for lexical development.

The sandtray therapy provides a needed and effective communication medium for individuals with poor verbal skills: people with social or relational difficulties, with physical deficits, or ones who use English as a second language. The therapy has a unique kinaesthetic quality, especially addressed to people with visual impairment, who are eager and motivated to be brought into mobility. The sandtray therapy provides this sensory experience and meets the need for kinaesthetic experiences. The very tactile experience of touching and manipulating sand is a therapeutic experience that reduces tension and anxiety (Kalff, 1980). It appears as if the sensory experience with sand causes "a loosening of the tongue". The manipulation of sand is safe and kinaesthetically satisfying, especially for those whose prior sensory experience was noxious.

The sandtray is a container for sand (Homeyer and Sweeney, 2011). A standard tray is rectangular with approximately 60 by 40cm and 7cm deep, made of wood or plastic. The rectangular shape facilitates dividing the sandtray scene into sections. It is certainly possible to have a tray that is in another shape, such as square, round, or octagonal. Also plant saucers of various sizes or restaurant take-out containers may provide a variety of options. The sand should fill about one half of the depth of the tray, which should be waterproof. It is also advisable to have two trays available, one wet and the other dry. There are distinct advantages to having water available. Like sand, water has a unique sensory and kinaesthetic quality, changing the consistency and malleability of the sand. Margaret Lowenfeld (1950: 329) commented upon this:

> Sand and water lend themselves to the demonstration of a large variety of fantasies. When wet, the sand may be moulded, and when dry it is pleasant to feel, and many tactile experiments can be made with the gradual addition of moisture.

There are various types of sand that can be used in the sandtray (Homeyer and Sweeney 2011). It is recommended to use sand that is not too coarse, which is often filled with small pebbles. It should be emphasised that rice and/or corn can also be added to sand. Small glass, plastic beads, miniatures or realia may be acceptable alternatives. Miniatures are objects, words, symbols that provide individuals with diverse vocabulary that can be arranged in different categories: people, animals, buildings, transportation, food, signs, natural items, fantasy, feelings, landscaping and other accessories, household items, and miscellaneous items. The categories should always be in the same place due to the on-going therapeutic need for consistency. Consistency promotes predictability, which promotes safety, especially in relation to visually impaired students.

Processing a scene in the sandtray may be an intensively powerful experience. Global processing exists through defined elements of the process structure: the title, a general explanation – describing a tray, discussing scenes.

Badenoch (2008) indicates that the use of the sandtray awakens and regulates the right-brain limbic processes, promoting vertical integration in the right brain. The sensations travel to the prefrontal cortex, which makes sense of tactile input. "When the individual recalls painful experiences and is met with empathy and kindness, new synapses carry that information throughout the brain and blood flow changes course to more soothing paths" (p. 12). Once the tray is created and verbally analysed, the content results in left and right brain integration. Adding words to the story, which occurs in the left brain, to the imagery and feelings of the right brain, actually strengthens the corpus callosum (the connecting tissue between the left and right hemispheres) resulting in greater regulation of the emotional content of the sandtray experience.

The choice to use sand as the foundation of the sandtray therapy was not accidental; it was a purposeful and intentional therapeutic intervention or technique in the PLT process.

The practical implication is presented in the empirical part (subchapter 5.3).

4.4. The Brain Linkage Method – Bioemanation (BSM)

I was trying to create a multisensory therapy that covers various aspects of the visually impaired development. As was said earlier, the PLT focuses on human mental development that is paralleled by the growing importance of language. That was the reason to apply the Brain Linkage Method (BSM) to support the process of achieving mental balance, overcoming stress, and improving concentration and memory for language and psyche involvement.

I have experienced the effects of the Brain Linkage Method on myself and on my son. Our brains are maps. This mapping results from the way connections in the brain are ordered and arranged. The ordering of neural pathways between different parts of the brain and those going to and from our muscles and sensory organs produces specific patterns on the brain surface that can be seen at various levels of organisation. At the most general level, areas that control motor functions (muscle movement) map to the front-most areas of the cerebral cortex, while areas that receive and process sensory information are more towards the back of the brain. Each sensory area is divided even further into a more detailed map. The sensory pathways from the skin, which give information on pain, temperature, and touch, are mapped onto the somatosensory cortex. This mapping of our sense of touch onto the cortex gives us a representation of the body, which was named the homunculus by Wilder Penfield (Penfield, 1975).

The figures below display the sensory areas on the frontal cross-section of the brain; they illustrate the cortical representation of various parts of the body (Chusid, 1996).

Figure 14. The sensory and motor homunculus in the forehead plane of the brain cross-section by Wider Penfield (after Lewandowski, 2005:20)

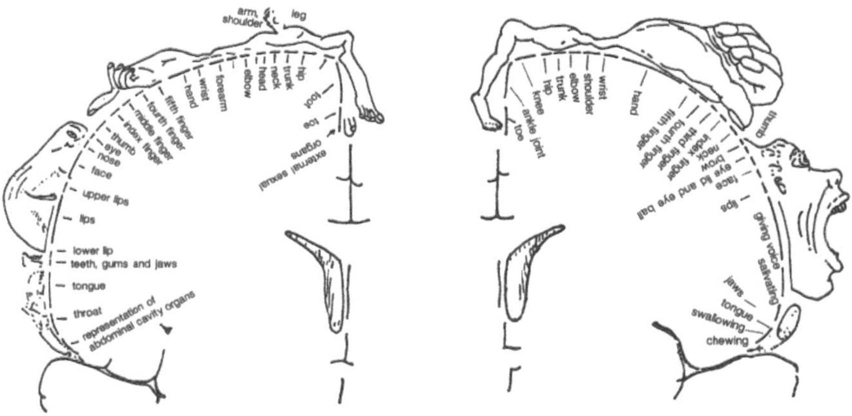

The size of each body region in the homunculus is related to the density of sensory receptors. The stimulation of various regions of the sensory or motor cortex produces tingling or movement in the part of the body (Penfield, 1975).

The Brain Linkage Method, based on Penfield's homunculus, is a method of self-healing and treatment for reinstating the body's internal balance, unsettled by the result of mental or physical disorders. BSM was discovered by Eugeniusz Uchnast. Bioemanation (the other name for BSM) is "all radiation emanated by an organism on the surface of the body of unrestricted scope of a diversity of forms" (Lewandowski, 2005:4). Distinct from other non-conventional therapies, the BSM method acts directly on the central nervous system, balancing the two hemispheres. Since that system is enormously sensitive to receiving weak electro-magnetic fields, the energy radiated by every person is sufficient (with palms or wrists put on the sensory zone-head), in varying degrees, to evoke healing reactions. This sensitivity is related to the presence of magnetic crystals in the human brain. In the BSM therapy, the central nervous system is "fed", and further, the changes in the organism's electromagnetic field are eliminated (Lewandowski, 2005).

Determination of the sense point

The key issue of the BSM therapy is to define the location of the sense point. For the purpose of determining the proper placement of palms, the auxiliary point called the "sense point" (Figure 15) has to be found on the skull. The distance should be measured from the "nasion" 0% point, between the eyebrows along the skull centre-line, to the "inion" 100%, the lowest bump on the back of the skull (cranial protuberance), which can be felt just above the top of the neck. The cranial point is situated halfway along that line. The "sense point" is located 3 cm further toward the back of the skull (occiput); using a measuring tape to define the "sense point" is recommended (Lewandowski 2005).

Figure 15. Topography of the brain in the skull (after Lewandowski, 2005:9)

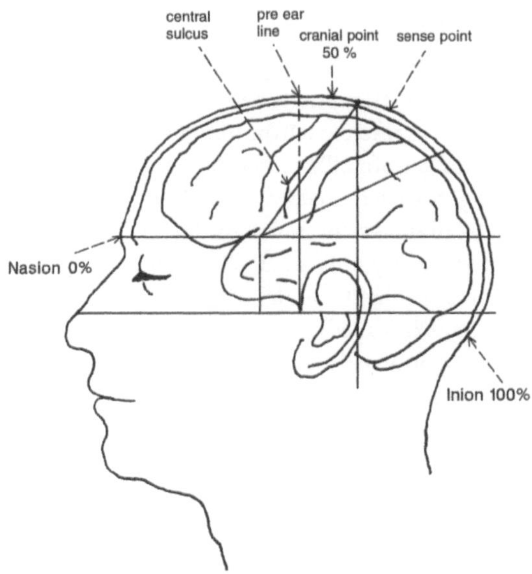

Auxiliary lines should be marked on the palms. One should run along the middle-finger axis, the second perpendicular to it, under the finger-joint pulvinars (palm transversal line). The point where they intersect is the conventional centre of the palm (Figure 16).

Figure 16. Lines displaying the skull centreline (after Lewandowski, 2005:12)

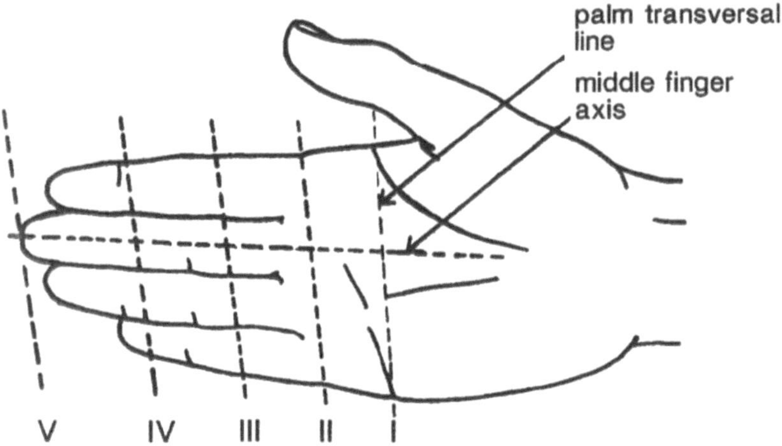

Treatment position issues

Muscled layers of the palm give off the greatest radiation – the balls of the small finger and thumb. The radiation emitted by the live cellular tissue of the hand arouses those centres to commence self-healing processes, on the selected site on the head responsible for certain afflicted parts of the body.

The palm, with fingers closed except for the thumb, should rest with its whole surface on the skull in all treatment positions. It should rest gently without great pressure being exerted. Both palms are used simultaneously. The middle fingers rest on the "sense point", in slight contact with each other. The palms are located at a slightly slanted angle. It makes no difference whether the person him/herself or another applies the treatment. The palm may be substituted by another part of the body, preferably a well-muscled part, for instance a forearm.

Healing procedures are often accompanied by piercing, burning, heating or cooling sensations, even pulsation of the palm or the skin on one's skull. The BSM method may not bring the expected results in the case of placing a palm improperly (Lewandowski 2005).

The practical implication is presented in the empirical part (subchapter 5.4).

4.5. Edu-kinaesthetic field

The brain is surely the most complex organ in the human body. Each of its two halves has unique properties. Although each half, or hemisphere, of the brain appears to be a mirror image of the other, there are both physical and functional differences. The left hemisphere generally governs speech and verbal reasoning. The right hemisphere, in contrast, bears responsibility for spatial visualisation, holistic thinking, face recognition, music perception, and perception of emotional expression (Chusid, 1996). Each side of the brain is associated with the opposite side of the body. Information provided by the left of the body is reported to the right hemisphere, and vice versa. The left hemisphere processes stimuli from the right half of the body and controls movement on one side. The left hemisphere, dominant for most people, controls such mental tasks as language. The right half is limited in its language capacity, but excels in the ability to recognise patterns and process spatial relationships. The connection between the hemispheres is vital for the communication of learning and memory (Bandler, 1985).

Language is not distributed equally between the two hemispheres. Moreover, within the left hemisphere it is located toward the front rather than toward the back. On the basis of "dichotic" listening tests, the right ear in adult humans is dominant for speech sounds. If in such tests either one set of digits is presented to one ear and a different set to the other, or one message is presented to one ear and a different one to the other ear, listeners will overwhelmingly report hearing what was presented to the right ear rather than to the left ear. But for tunes presented in this way the favoured ear will be the left one. It may even be that the left side of the brain is responsible not only for language but also for other "higher intellectual" processes too, e.g. reasoning. On the other hand, the right side of the brain is said to be "visually-spatially" oriented so that its "preference" is for non-speech sound, music, melody, and perhaps even emotional expression. So lateralisation of the brain may extend well beyond language alone (Wardhaugh, 1994).

I chose the edu-kinaesthetic area (brain gym), not only to establish the "waterfall" of positive feelings, but also to reinforce relaxation, and to focus on practising concentration and memory to stimulate the effective coordination within the two hemispheres of the brain of my visually impaired students.

Kinaesthetic dance or brain gym is associated with Paul Dennison, the discoverer of the "brain gym". The brain gym programme provides a series of simple movement activities that optimise brain activity, while integrating the mind and body (Dennison, 2003). They also focus on seeing a positive result, which is a driving force for continuing to do them on a regular basis. The kinaesthetic awareness of the space of one's body is the core of Dennison's movement (Hannaford, 1998).

Summing up, the students have learnt to trust their bodies, with an emphasis put on the awareness of the body.

The practical implication is depicted in the empirical study (subchapter 5.5).

Part Two: Empirical Part

Chapter Five: Practical implications of the psycho-linguistic therapy "Touching the World"

5.0. Introductory remarks

Chapter five presents practical implications of the psycho-linguistic therapy "Touching the World", especially the core consideration of the thesis – the Re-charged Direct Method. It also combines the sandtray therapy, Bioemanation, and "brain gym" with appropriate classroom arrangements issues. Useful and creative techniques, based on sensory compensation, are shown within "tactile structure repetition".

5.1. The PLT steps division

The PLT covers 74 sessions (the figure below) that are recognised within two categories of steps. In the "Touching the World" therapy definite steps are distinguished: *pre-steps*, that work in correlation with Relaxed Feedbacks covering 6 sessions; and *proper steps*: 1 and 2 of Re-charged Water and Re-charged Collage Feedbacks, which incorporate 68 sessions. Each proper step correlates within 34 sessions on the PLT issues with a difference of evaluations: 2 (step 1) or 3 (step 2).

Figure 17. The PLT steps division

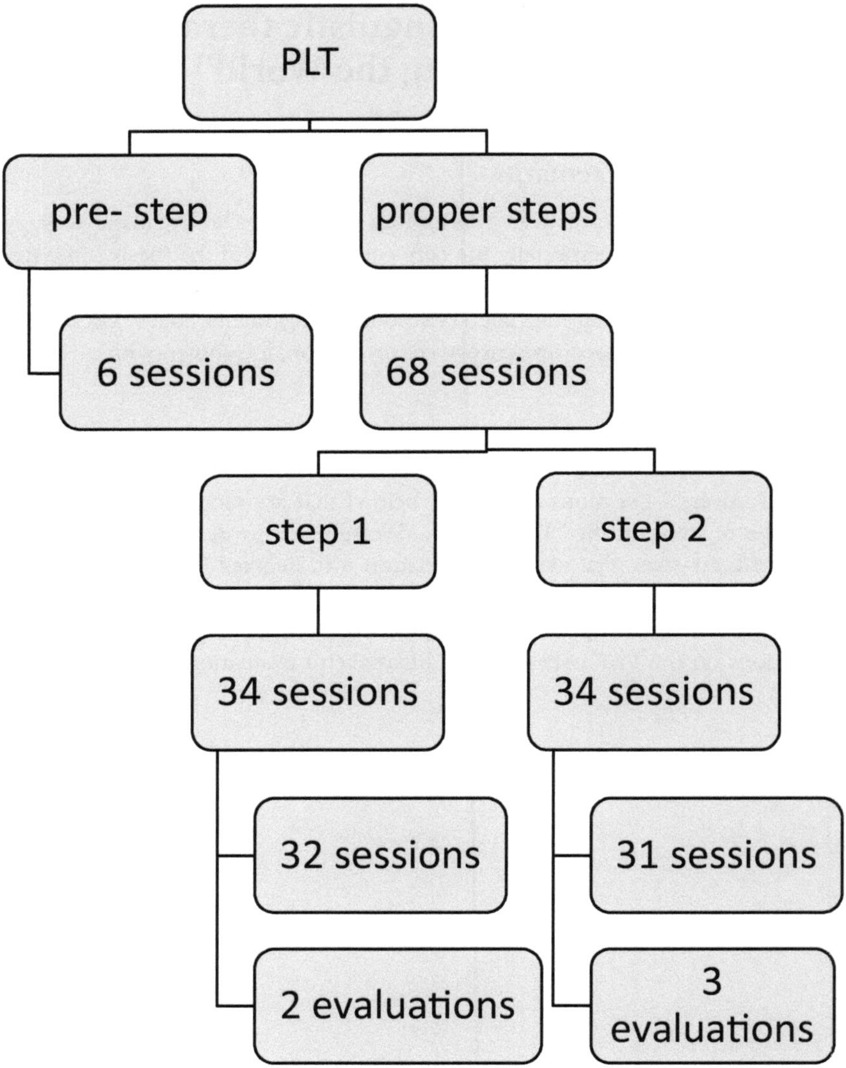

5.2. The Re-charged Direct Method

The cluster lasts about 38–40 minutes with the predominance of 20-minute speaking comprehension as the core issue of the Re-charged Direct Method, then 4-second acquisition, taking 8 minutes, and parallel reading or dicto-listening, limited to about 10-minute involvements (Figure 18).

Both Re-charged Collage Feedback and Re-charged Water Feedback incorporate the Re-charged Direct Method as a basis for linguistic development.

Figure 18. The Re-charged Direct Method structure

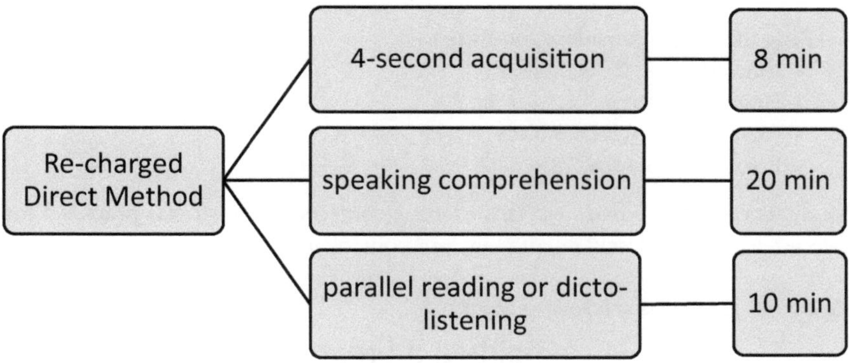

The structure of the Re-charged Direct Method

STAGE I.

4-second acquisition is incorporated in the controlled breathing cluster, which is divided into the pre-controlled breathing and controlled breathing (depicted in subchapter 4.2.1.).

The rhythmic breathing procedure during the ***pre-controlled breathing*** (Figure 19):

(1) The first practice supplies the step to achieve the rhythmic breath; students count to 4, on every stage of the task.
- Inhalation – 1,2,3,4
- Holding a breath – 1,2,3,4
- Exhalation – 1,2,3,4
- Break – 1,2,3,4

They repeat it four times. Then they concentrate on the second task.

(2) The second breathing task; the same rule, but counting is different – students count to 6.
- Inhalation – 1,2,3,4,5,6
- Holding a breath – 1,2,3,4,5,6
- Exhalation – 1,2,3,4,5,6
- Break – 1,2,3,4,5,6

They repeat it four times. Then they continue breathing practice with the third task.

(3) The third type considers counting to 8.
- Inhalation – 1,2,3,4,5,6,7,8
- Holding a breath – 1,2,3,4,5,6,7,8
- Exhalation – 1,2,3,4,5,6,7,8
- Break – 1,2,3,4,5,6,7,8

Students repeat it four times. This exercise controls breath. It was practised for two weeks, twice a week, during four pre-controlled breath sessions.

Figure 19. The process of breathing practice

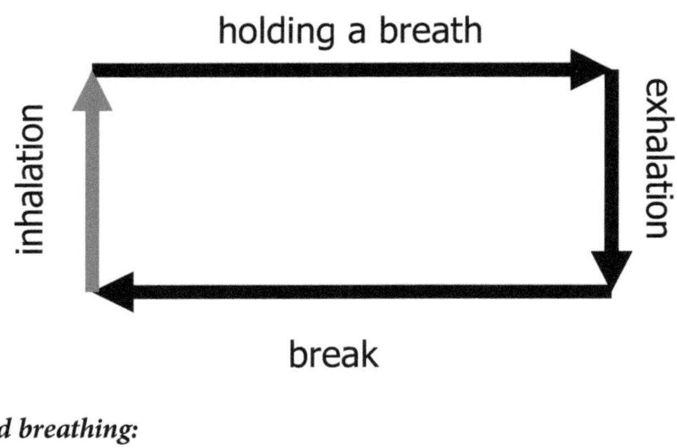

Controlled breathing:

The following pattern of 4-second acquisition (new material presentation):

(1) <u>the empty cycle</u> – only breathing (Figure 20)
- Inhalation – 4s
- Holding a breath – 4s
- Exhalation – 4s
- Break – 4s

Figure 20. Controlled breathing – the empty cycle rotation

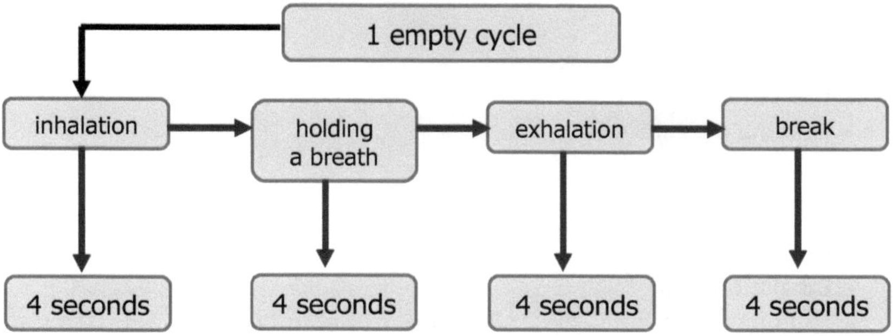

(2) <u>the primary cycle</u> (Figure 21)
- Inhalation – 4s
- Holding a breath – "*Where do you live?/ Where do you live?*" – 4s (the question is repeated by the teacher)
- Exhalation – 4s
- Break – 4s

(3) <u>the secondary cycle</u> (Figure 21)
- Inhalation – 4s
- Holding a breath – "*Where do you live?/ Where do you live?*"– 4s (the second repetition of the question)
- Exhalation – 4s
- Break – 4s

Figure 21. 4-second acquisition process – the primary/secondary rotation

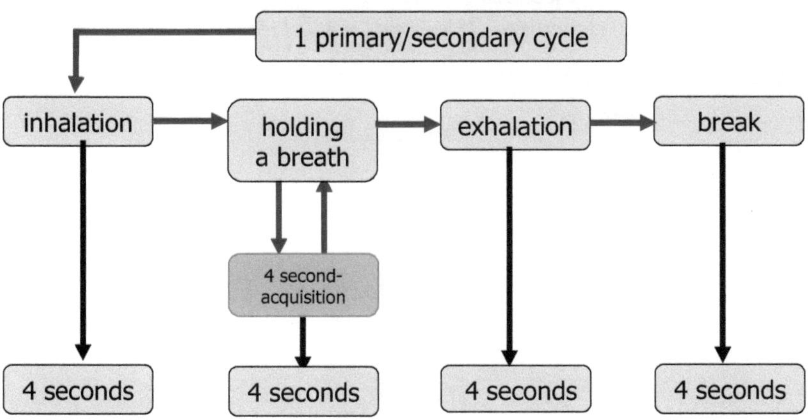

And again the same 4-second acquisition process **but** with an emphasis on a new structure:

(1) the empty cycle – only breathing
- Inhalation – 4s
- Holding a breath – 4s
- Exhalation – 4s
- Break – 4s

(2) the primary cycle
- Inhalation – 4s
- Holding a breath – "*I live in Bialystok. / I live in Bialystok.*" – 4s (the statement is repeated by the teacher)
- Exhalation – 4s
- Break – 4s

(3) the secondary cycle
- Inhalation – 4s
- Holding a breath – "*I live in Bialystok. / I live in Bialystok.*"– 4s (the second repetition of the statement)
- Exhalation – 4s
- Break – 4s

The form of the circle is segmental, with definite time issues given, and the number of repeated structures (Figures 22 and 23):

1. *1 phase* = 4 seconds
2. *1 cycle* = 4 phases · 4 seconds = 16 seconds
3. *1 circle* = 3 cycles · 16 seconds = 48 seconds = 1 structure
4. *10 structures* = 10 structures · 48 seconds = 480 seconds = 8 minutes

10 structures = 10 circles = 30 cycles = 8 minutes

Figure 22. 4-second acquisition – time schedule

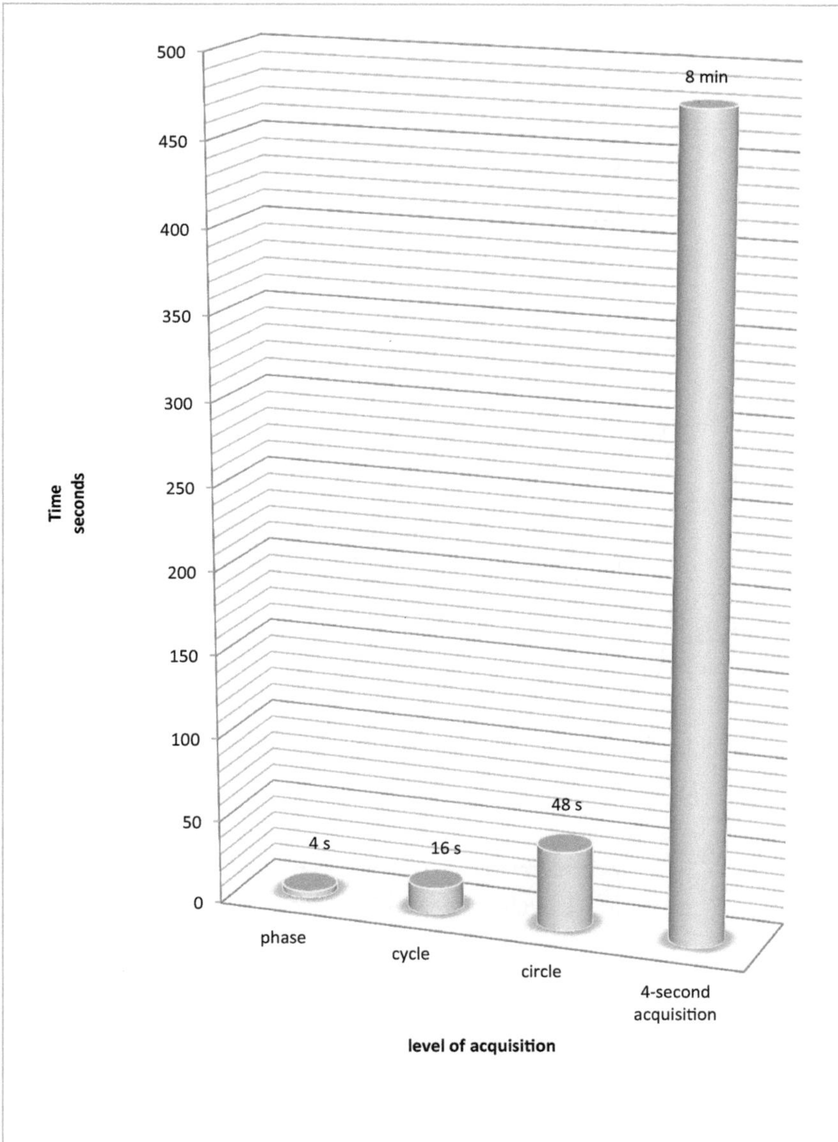

Figure 23. The 4-second acquisition process; one circle's time schedule

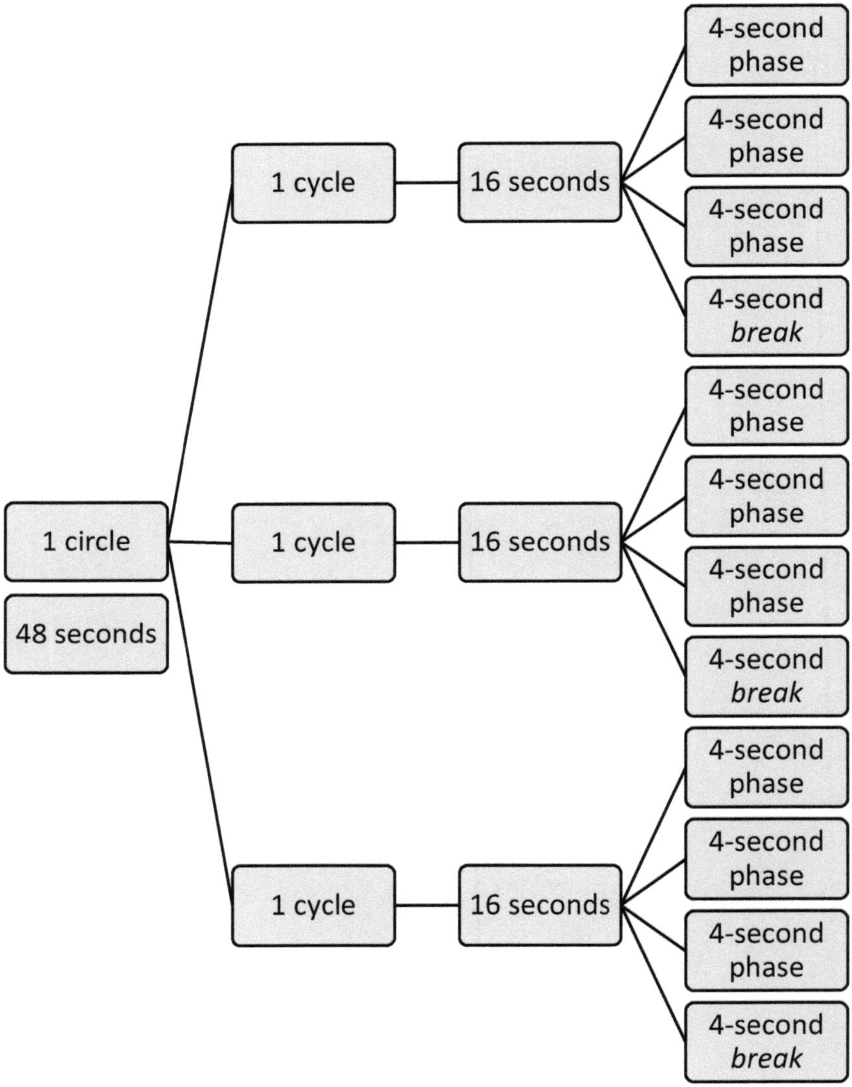

STAGE II.
Speaking comprehension – focuses on a teacher-student interaction – question-answer work, based upon 4-second acquisition programme.

Every question is repeated twice – based on the Callan Method (1995).

Example:

Teacher: *Where do you live?*
Where do you live?

Student 1: *I live in Bialystok.*

Teacher: *Where do you live?*
Where do you live?

Student 2: *I live in Bialystok.*

Teacher: *Do you live in a city or in the country?*
Do you live in a city or in the country?

Student 3: *I live in a city. etc…*

STAGE III.
Dicto-listening or parallel reading – students practise the same question-answer work (implemented in segment 1–4-second acquisition, and segment 2 – speaking comprehension) within procedures described in subchapter 4.2.2.

5.3. The sandtray therapy

Conducting a sandtray session focuses on some crucial steps (Sweeney, 1999):

- *Stage one:* setting up a room.
- *Stage two:* introducing the sandtray therapy – individuals may be given a directive or nondirective approach, or both. Giving minimal or no directions allows the scene to be a result of the person's interaction with sand.

The favourite use of the sandtray is directed to creating trays with the following instructions:

(1) covering the mental layer of the PLT – *Make a scene in sand that shows your feelings about your family, home, work, about being … visually impaired etc.* or just focusing on students' nondirective creation.
(2) covering the linguistic layer of the PLT – *Make a scene in sand that answers the question or describes a thematic field:*

- *"Where do you live?"*
- *"What's your hobby?"*
- *"Build a place where you'd like to live."*
- *"Prepare your favourite salad."*
- *"In a shop …"– dicto-listening focus.*
- *"Create your English classroom."*
- *"My room is …"*
- *"What is your favourite season of the year?"*
- *"What job would you like to take in the future?"*
- *"Your family tree …"*
- *"Giving directions" – dicto-listening focus.*
- *"In the kitchen …" etc.*

– *Stage three:* the creation stage – the individuals build the scenes in the sandtray, developing and maintaining the therapeutic environment in which a person does verbally his or her work. The individual must believe, know, think, and feel that he or she is emotionally and physically safe.
The product – the completed tray – is obviously salient. At the same time, observing the individual's process is paramount. The area of observation during the process of building the sandtray is how a person interacts with media, developing his/her linguistic competences (De Domenico, 1995):
  > Does he/she spend a great deal of time smoothing and resmoothing the surface?
  > Is the sand moved about, piled up here, exposing the bottom of the box there?
  > In damp sand, are tunnels made?
  > Does a person carefully make sure not to touch the sand at all?
  > Does a person avoid certain objects or categories?
  > Does a person speak English: using separate words, phrases or sentences?

– *Stage four:* the postcreation phase. The scene in the sandtray works as a springboard for the discussion and continued verbal work with a person. People often discover insights for themselves regardless of whether it was a directed or non-directed experience.

– *Stage five:* documenting the sandtray session.
The sandtray description (a session form – Appendix B) includes definite words and expressions that depict students' sandtrays: one idea, several ideas, wet, dry, organised, chaotic, open, closed, empty, excessive, rigid, realistic, dynamic, static, peaceful, aggressive, buried, purposeful, nonpurposeful, determined, hesitant, unpeopled, people, verbal, non-verbal.

5.4. The Brain Linkage Method

During the PLT sessions positions V and I were involved. The choice of treatment positions implies the goals of the therapy, leading to the development of better memory and concentration, and general-mental balance.

BSM time indicators

Each BSM method procedure lasts from 15 to 20 minutes. The first session should be prolonged to 35 minutes, then about a half-hour break, and again 20 minutes of radiation, then once again the same break and a 20-minute treatment. This is the first beginning session schedule.

Treatment position I (Lewandowski, 2005)

Figure 24 presents the cross-section of the brain with a visible gap between the hemispheres. This gap is covered in position 1 as a result of which the vegetative system is primarily acted upon. This system is divided into the parasympathetic and sympathetic nervous system (Altman, 1970).

Figure 24. Diagram of a human cerebral cortex (after Altman 1970, in Lewandowski 2005:21)

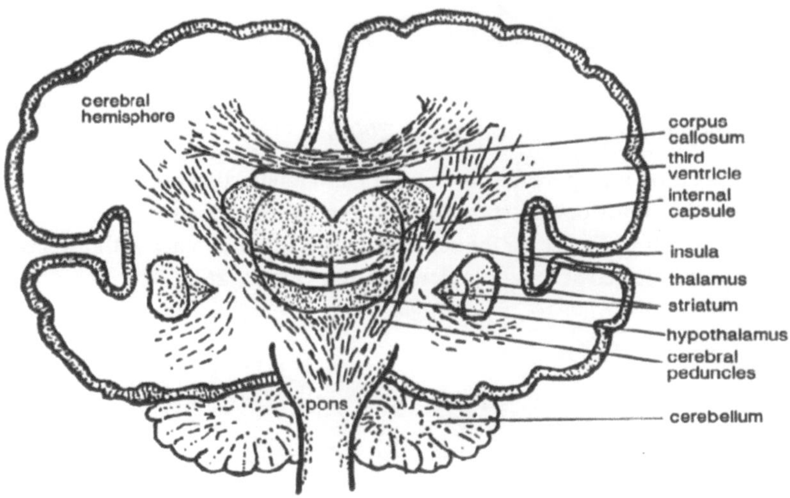

This position influences mental equilibrium and neurosis.

The palm should be placed on the skull so that the centre of the palm coincides with the skull "sense point". The palm transversal line should simultaneously coincide with the skull centre line. The thumb should be spread, the remaining fingers held together so that the whole surface of the fingers is in contact with the skull (Figure 25).

Figure 25. Treatment position 1 (after Lewandowski, 2005:11)

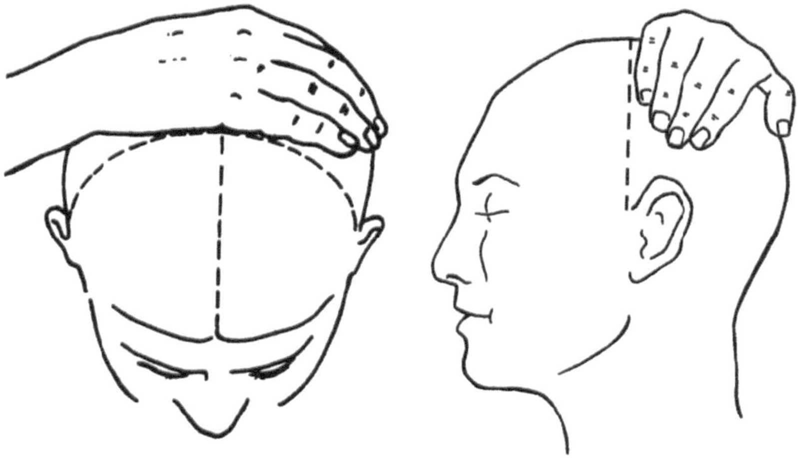

Treatment position V (Lewandowski, 2005)

The fifth position is responsible for memory and intellectual proficiency and also focuses on the ability of concentration and overcoming stress.

The middle fingers rest on the sense point, in slight contact with each other. The palms are located at a slightly slanted angle (Figure 26).

Figure 26. Treatment position 5 (after Lewandowski, 2005:14)

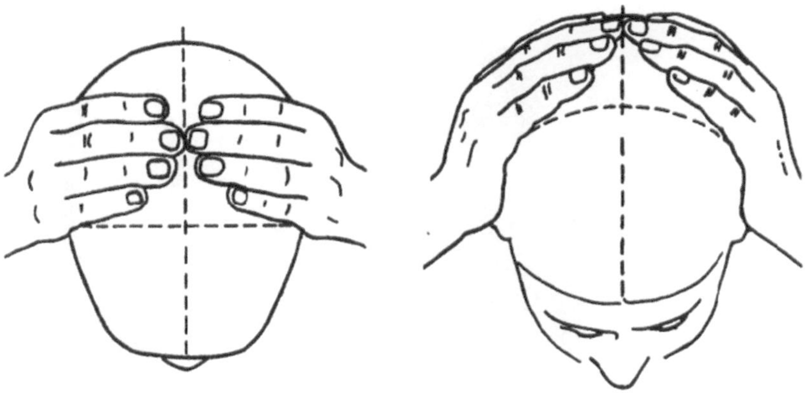

In essence, development of mental balance, better concentration, and memory improvement were influenced by Bioemanation support, leading to achievements in L2.

5.5. Edu-kinaesthetic field

These are the following activities (Dennison, 2003; Hannaford, 1998) performed to achieve an emotional balance approach, in the order of appearance in the PLT "Touching the World":

Lazy 8s (Figure 27) – a student aligns his/her body with a point at the eye level; this will be the midpoint of the 8. A person draws the lazy 8s adjusting the width and height to fit his/her needs. He/she starts on the midline and moves counter-clockwise first, up, over, and around; then from his/her waist he/she moves clockwise, up, over, around and back to the beginning of the midpoint. The head moves slightly and the neck remains relaxed. The exercise was repeated with each hand separately and then both together; it provides a relaxation process.

Figure 27. Edu-kinaesthetic crossing the centre body line (lazy 8s)

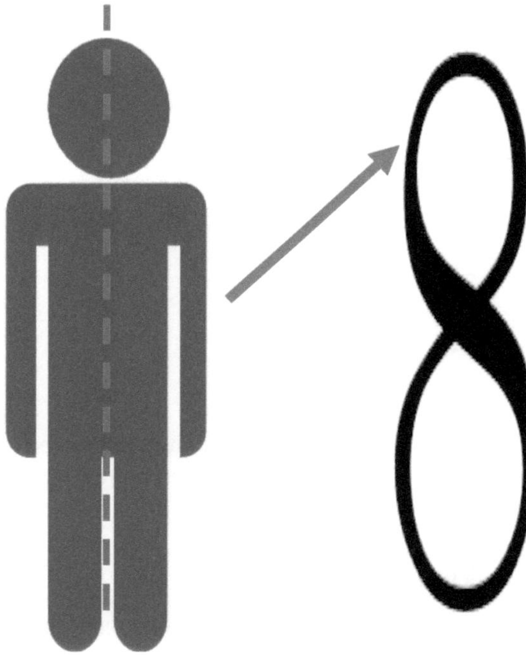

Cross-crawl – simultaneously a person lifts his/her right hand and left leg, lightly tapping the hand just above his/her left knee; then he/she returns the hand and leg to a resting position as he/she lifts his/her left hand and right leg, touching his/her left hand to the place above the opposite knee. Then he/she continues this back and forth pattern for a minute or so, as though walking rhythmically. This improves left-right coordination; it helps with concentration and supports the respiratory system and stamina.

Positive points – a person lightly touches the points above each eye, halfway between eyebrows and the hairline, with the fingertips of each hand; using just enough pressure to pull the skin taut and holding the contact for about a minute are the issues of this exercise. It helps with speaking skills.

Arm activation – a person reaches up above the head with the left arm, feeling the arm lengthen from the rib cage. This works as the first step. The next step is holding the arm just below the elbow with the right hand, followed by the isometric activation of the left arm for a few seconds in each of four positions away from the head, forward, backward, and toward the ear. A person rests his/her arm again at his/her side. Now the person stands and lets his/her arms hang comfortably by his/her sides. This improves focus and concentration without the focus itself; it also improves breathing and a relaxed attitude.

The brain gym takes 5 minutes during the PLT and appears during 63 sessions, with the activities practised interchangeably, during Re-charged Collage Feedback (described in subchapter 5.6.2.), with the involvement of "lazy 8s" and "cross-crawls". The exercises "positive points" and "arm activation" appear in Re-charged Water Feedback (subchapter 5.6.3.).

5.6. Feedbacks involvement

The PLT consists of three feedbacks: Relaxed, Re-charged Collage and Re-charged Water that are closely related to the Re-charged Direct Method; they work as supportive tools.

5.6.1. Relaxed Feedback

Relaxed Feedback is devoted to the analysis of individual psychological blockers that need to be diminished or balanced through diverse segmental issues of the therapy.

The feedback consists of four sessions:

Session 1 covers the discussion zone lasting 30 minutes, then a 5-minute edu-kinaesthetic area appears, then students breathe in a controlled way during the pre-controlled breath cluster, which takes 15 minutes; then a 10-minute break before the longest module of Bioemanation. It is advisable to linger on the first BSM radiation for up to 35 minutes in the first contact session.

During the session, the predominant segment correlates with the Brain Linkage Method. The discussion zone time aspect grows almost in parallel with the Bioemanation time rate (Figure 28A).

Sessions 2–4 differ from session 1 just in one element of the Brain Linkage Method (it takes 20 minutes). Other segments still present the same time parameters. The discussion zone prevails, according to the therapy aims. Sessions 2–4 last 80 minutes, considering the time difference between the first and next Brain Linkage Method sessions (Figure 28B).

Figure 28A. The length of the Relaxed Feedback structure – session 1

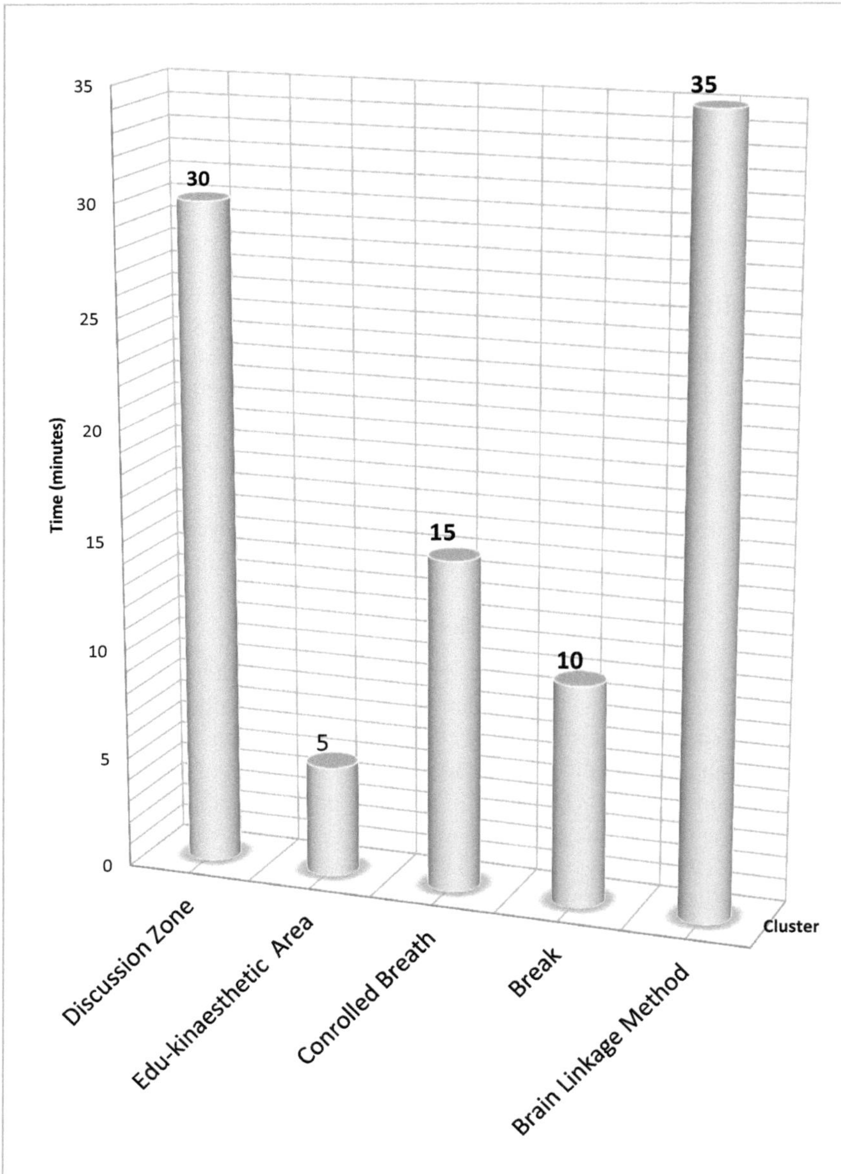

Figure 28B. The length of the Relaxed Feedback structure – sessions 2–4

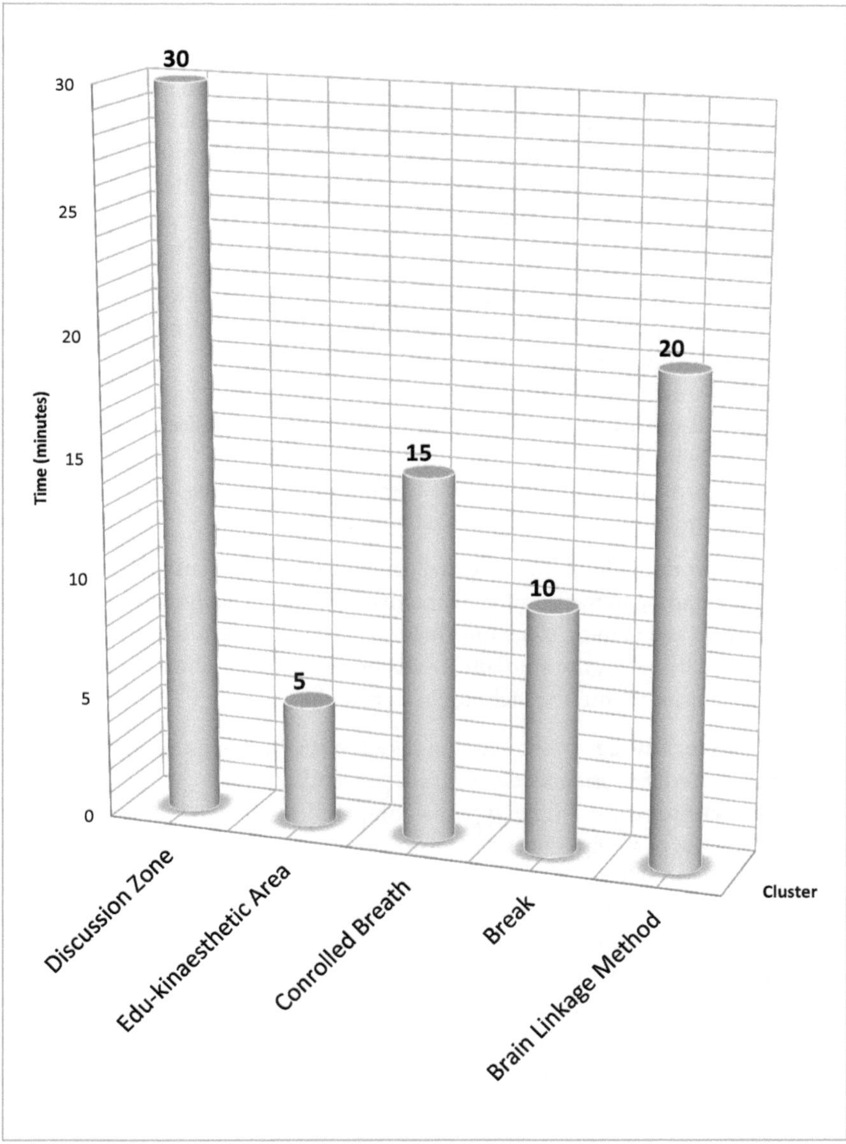

Discussion zone

The discussion zone module is incorporated in Relaxed Feedback, with an analysis of psychological blockers. The module leads to awakening the awareness of destructive feelings the students shared, and then focuses on an increase in positive affects (interested, excited, strong, enthusiastic, proud, alert, inspired, determined, attentive, active), and a decrease in negative affects (afraid, distressed, upset, guilty, scared, hostile, irritable, ashamed, nervous and jittery).

The formation of each of four sessions is related to diverse emotions the students elaborated on. It lasts 30 minutes.

Session 1 – combines the element-consequence of the visual impairment such as a pain-fear distractor, with the issue "without our control" and "within our control".
Session 2 – emits resentment, hatred, criticism, and anger.
Session 3 – discusses problems of depression, guilt, confusion, hence asking "why questions".
Session 4 – aims at activating defence mechanisms, with the aspect of time – the future, present, and past analyses.

Each session works within a **4d's rule** that defines the steps: **d**iscuss, **d**estroy, **d**ance, and **d**iscover leading to overcoming distractive feelings – negative affects, developing self-esteem and gaining some information of the awareness of the body.

During the first step, the students discussed mental distractors, crucial in *self development* tasks, within the techniques I created:

- **Spaghetti technique** – a comparison between *raw* and *boiled* spaghetti; raw – a tense, scared person, boiled – relaxed, peaceful.
- **Apple technique** – a whole apple is compared to the past: "swallowing" is accepting the past; pips cover the future; the process of eating an apple is the present – "eating life".
- **Billa technique** – physical movement of a plastic ball, tied on ropes or a string to emphasise the intensity of emotions shared with others.
- **Balloon technique** consists of pejorative emotions that are blown into balloons by the students during each of four sessions.
- **Lego blocks technique** – the students build individual emotional towers; one block expresses one feeling.

Then the individuals were asked to treat the emotions as rubbish; their task was focused on crumpling sheets of paper (compared with blockers), and throwing them out into a "negative feeling dustbin"; anger, pain, loneliness, all the feelings that stopped their growth were "physically destroyed". The next element of this cluster appeared on the basis of the previous ones. The students danced, moved, or "waved" their bodies within "emotional dance", with the background music playing; the aim was related to the achievement of the acceptance of self (Figure 29).

Figure 29. The discussion zone – 4 d's rule

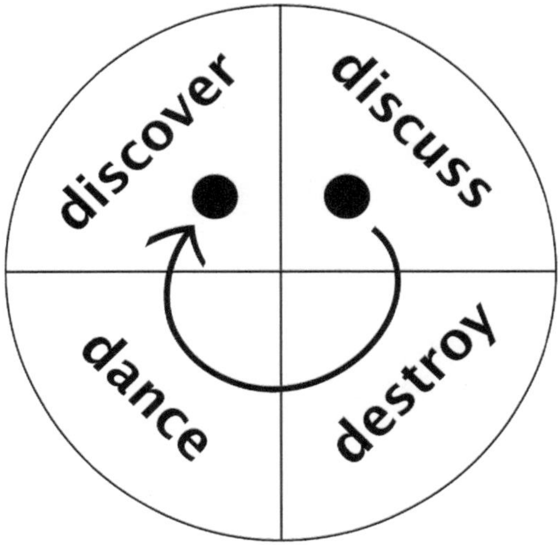

In essence, language itself opens through various vivid techniques, through the awareness of self-esteem and self-acceptance, with a noticeable, creative reciprocation.

5.6.2. Re-charged Collage Feedback

Re-charged Collage Feedback aims at teaching-learning lexis. The structure of the feedback comprises the 20-minute Brain Linkage Method cluster, limited to position 1, and the controlled breathing area, lasting 5 minutes, as initial points. The feedback focuses on the 40-minute Re-charged Direct Method, enriched with 4-second acquisition practice, speaking comprehension and dicto-listening; then a 5-minute break and 5-minute appearance of the edu-kinaesthetic field. The core issue is the 30-minute collage support related to lexical engagement and, finally, the discussion zone field, taking 10 minutes, which joins all segments in one added value. The feedback lasts 120 minutes (Figure 30).

Figure 30. The Re-charged Collage Feedback structure

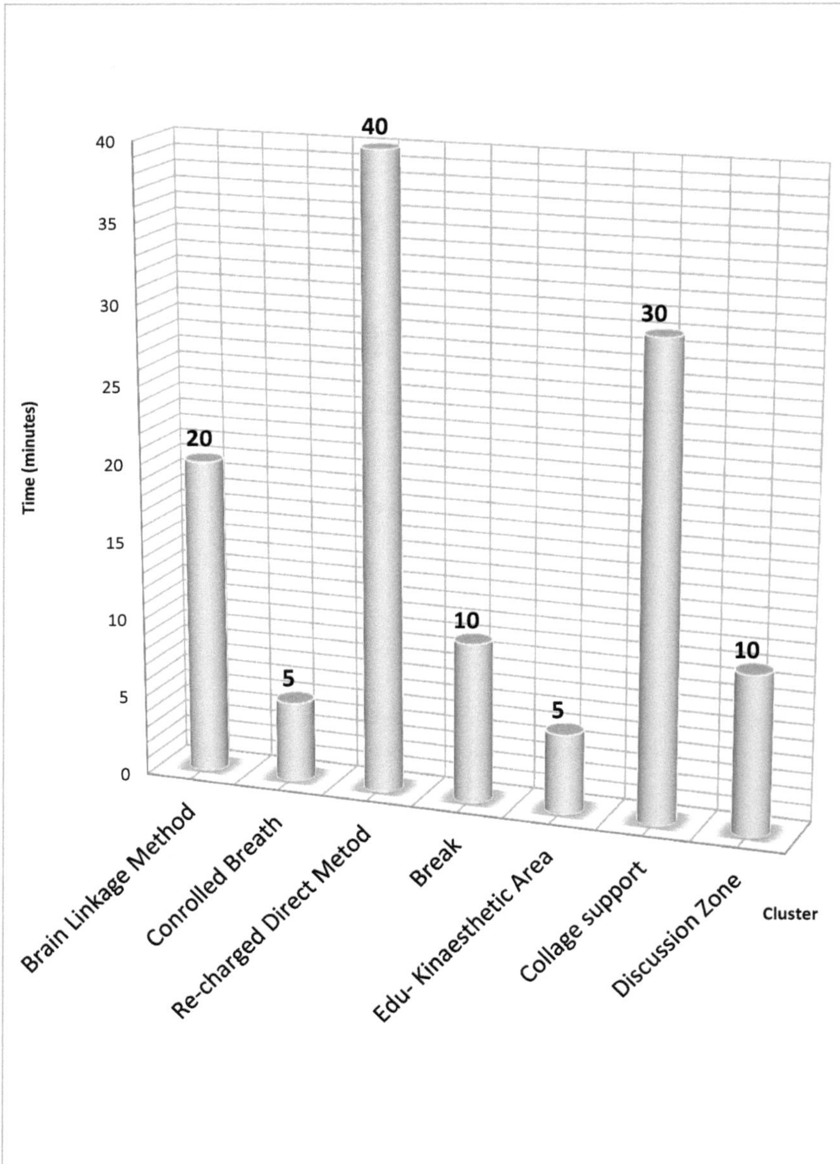

Collage support

The crucial aspect of the research was correlated with vocabulary that needs to be recycled to be learnt; the expanding recycling is the core issue of the psycho-language therapy, with gradually increasing intervals (Baddeley, 1983). The cluster puts an emphasis on the plurality of tactile-audible repetitions. The revision of words is employed in the multiple repetition chain that involves the pattern: after 15 minutes, 2 days, 1 week, 1 month and 2 months.

The collage support lasts 30 minutes once a week and covers 32 vocabulary sessions per school year; it is directly related to teaching-learning vocabulary through the usage of sensory compensation techniques. I utilised the compensation of the remaining senses to make the process creative, communicatively effective and involving appropriate tasks that activate sensory compensation mechanisms.

The following lexical areas were involved in the PLT process:

Introductions, emotions, classroom, numbers, days of the week, months, seasons, colours, hobbies, telling the time, clothes, countries and nationalities, parts of the body, giving directions, house, food, man, family, jobs, shopping, health, entertainment.

I was trying to put the word fields in a bizarre, but (crucially) well-organised way, easy to be acquired. I emphasise a wide variety of ways in which the vocabulary chains were built to facilitate the learning process, focusing on tactile perception involvement, with the awareness that touch recognises words-objects, first their textures and then shapes. I tried not to teach words that were very similar in order to avoid becoming cross-associated in the learners' minds. Words that are strongly associated with each other, such as antonyms, were more difficult to learn together than words that have weak connections, or no relationship at all. I also focused on word pairs that appeared to be an effective tool for giving initial exposure to new words. Knowing that a word entails more than one meaning, lexis was always put in context (Morgan and Rinvolucri, 1997).

Within the sphere of lexis, I created various teaching-learning English techniques (except the sandtray therapy, described in subchapters 4.3. and 5.3):

(1) *Vocabulary movement (word segmentation)*, is a group work technique used for teaching lexis during Re-charged Collage Feedback sessions. Word segmentation focuses on the efficient activation of the kinaesthetic deficit of the visually impaired through speaking comprehension that is in movement. Vocabulary movement employs the whole body in physical and linguistic cooperation in a mechanical, dependent way. The technique is involved in

the lexical layer of recognition, being the support for the acquisition of polysyllabic and difficult words.

This correlates with the expression "words in steps". Each step is devoted to one word. The step is divided into sub-steps, depending on the length of the word. A sub-step is a part of a step, done in a slow pace. Each sub-step incorporates one syllable of the word. The rhythm of each step indicates the division of the word into syllables. The movement involves students going straight on, revising loudly the same word a few times with diverse speed combinations based on the word length, and with the last syllable-sub-step put physically on the ground, placing an emphasis on the end of the last pronounced syllable of the word. The process of "step development" begins with two-syllable words. Each step is emphasised by the sound of a rattle to make word segmentation vivid and rhythmical. Each word is depicted by the amount of syllables included and the rhythm itself.

An alternative to the word segmentation technique is back-chaining used in teaching oral language skills. The teacher pronounces the last syllable, the student repeats, and then the teacher continues, working backwards from the end of the word to the beginning, but enriched with the kinaesthetic activation of the body.

Summing up, a word is becoming a movement, which makes language learning kinaesthetically vivid and orally effective.

(2) *Aluminium foil technique* – focused on tactile pictures creation (related to individual work).
(3) *Taste a word technique* – students taste food trying to recognise words on the basis of taste (pair work involvement).
(4) *Billa technique* – physical movement of a plastic ball, tied on a string or ropes, moving along them, created for word formation tasks (pair work cooperation).

The following supportive teaching aids were implemented in the PLT process:

- wikki stix – flexible strips/threads that adhere to almost any smooth surface, with just fingertip pressure; reusable strips can be bent, moulded or just shaped to form creative tactile pictures.
- scented marker pens – watercolour marker pens with chisel tips; each colour represents a different smell.

In conclusion, the form of the teaching learning process within the PLT emits various types of empowerment: individual, pair, or group work.

5.6.3. Re-charged Water Feedback

Re-charged Water Feedback was used to create the sphere that teaches grammar through water experiments. The feedback is consolidated with the 40-minute Re-charged Direct Method, and the 30-minute water support, engaged in the grammar territory. Then an emphasis is put on Bioemanation, lasting 20 minutes, with the usage of treatment position 5, which leads to the 5-minute controlled breathing involvement through the 4-second acquisition process, supported with parallel reading, meeting the 5-minute discussion zone that estimates the feedback achievement. After 65 minutes students have a 10-minute break and afterwards they practise the 5-minute brain gym. The feedback lasts 120 minutes (Figure 31).

Figure 31. The Re-charged Water Feedback structure

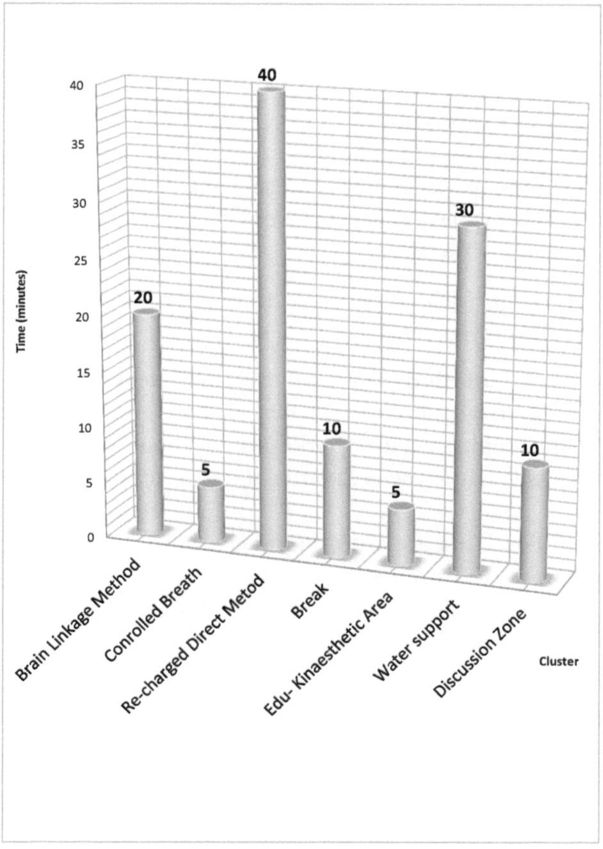

Water support

The water cluster is devoted to teaching-learning grammar issues through water techniques. The support is limited to five tenses to focus on: Present Continuous, Present Simple, Past Simple, Present Perfect and Future Simple. This mixture of tenses appears to be the basis of communicative language acquisition. Grammar issues are enriched with modal verbs (can, must), plurals of nouns, comparative and superlative adjectives, countable/uncountable nouns, and articles. The grammar field is taught through "ladder segments". One tense-segment is a rank for the next.

Grammar areas are correlated with a definite number of sessions.

The timetable of grammar issues for 31 sessions:

- Present Continuous – 4 sessions
- Present Simple/modal verbs – 4 sessions
- Simple Past – 4 sessions
- Future Simple – 2 sessions
- Present Perfect – 4 sessions
- Plural of nouns/articles – 2 sessions
- Comparative and superlative forms – 2 sessions
- Countable/uncountable nouns – 2 sessions
- Revision of tenses – 7 sessions

I discovered my own teaching grammar techniques, based on water, air, and kinaesthetic-tactile movement:

➢ **Grammar water jar technique** is used to establish tenses that "flow or sink in water". Three layers of grammatical issues are employed in the technique:
   1. The Future Simple structure – asking a question of an object that is held in the student's hands (before putting it into a jar of water): "Will it sink or float?"
   2. Then, if it floats, the Present Continuous comes into consideration, with the statement: "It is floating".
   3. Next, if the object does not float, the Present Perfect module appears: "It has sunk" (Figure 32).

Grammar structures covered in this technique: Future Simple, Present Continuous, Present Perfect.

Figure 32. Grammar water jar

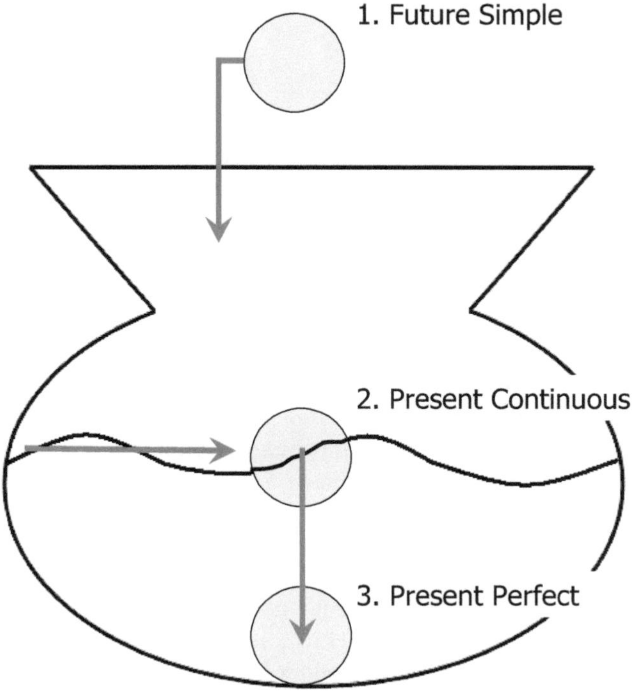

- **Water bottles technique** with different degrees of warmth that supports the tense recognition practice.

Grammar structures covered in this technique: Present Simple, Present Perfect, Past Simple, comparative and superlative forms.

- **Air technique** with the use of a hairdryer.

Grammar structures covered in this technique: Present Continuous, Present Perfect, comparative and superlative forms.

- **Billa technique** – a plastic ball tied on two strings that flies/moves from one person to the other; such movement accompanies loud sentence or word/phrases utterances.

Grammar structures covered in this technique: Present Simple, Present Continuous, Present Perfect, Past Simple, Future Simple, countable/uncountable nouns, plural of nouns, comparative and superlative forms, modal verbs, articles.

Water support cooperates with other tactile tasks, implemented in the grammar-layered acquisition within tactile structure repetition – TSR (analysed in the next subchapter).

5.7. Tactile structure repetition

The tactile structure repetition (TSR) is a multi-layered tool I designed to use for grammar and lexis repetitions. As the name itself indicates, not only is audible repetition practice required, but, in the aspect of teaching the visually impaired, haptic involvement is predominantly salient.

Tactile grammar cooperates with ping-pong sentence structures, tactile knots, and the sentence magnetic system (considered below).

It is worth emphasising that such a plurality of tactile-audible practice builds efficient language teaching.

Grammar structures covered in these techniques: Present Simple, Present Continuous, Present Perfect, Past Simple, Future Simple, countable/uncountable nouns, plural of nouns, comparative and superlative forms, modal verbs.

➢ **The ping-pong sentence structure**

I was inspired by the ping-pong ball to compare it to sentence structure as a whole, built in one coherent ball segment. The students ought to feel the sentence structure through active touch in order to construct it properly. They should be aware of the parts of the sentence that work in a well-organised chain of occurrence, based on the proper sequence of appearance with the comprehensible division of the parts of the sentence employed in English: subject, predicate, object, with an added category for auxiliary verbs (Figure 33B). These three parts of the sentence correlate with ping-pong balls; two of them are cut into four halves. Each of three halves is shaped with a certain hole or incision that is related to a diverse part of the sentence, and one has no cut (Figure 33A). Only a predicate works as a whole ball; it stays as a basis that is covered with other halves assembled in the creation of a one-ball segment.

The sentence design focuses on putting the proper halves and the whole ball into a single piece. The properly-built sentence appears as one complex ping-pong ball; in the case of improper structure plateau, no cohesive ball emerges. Diverse types of sentences are employed in TSR tasks: affirmative and negative statements, and questions (Figure 33C).

The option for the balls' location is to make them glued to the surface with blu-tack during the sentence formation process.

The act of building the whole ball-structure joins speaking comprehension with the involvement of tactile perception. Each half of the ping-pong ball is fixed with a parallel utterance.

In essence, I would like to pay attention to the need for haptic impressions in the grammar presentation, practice, and production process, appearing in coherence with a speaking skill, with an emphasis put on the kinaesthetic movement of a structure itself within active touch development.

Figure 33A. The ping-pong balls – triple division

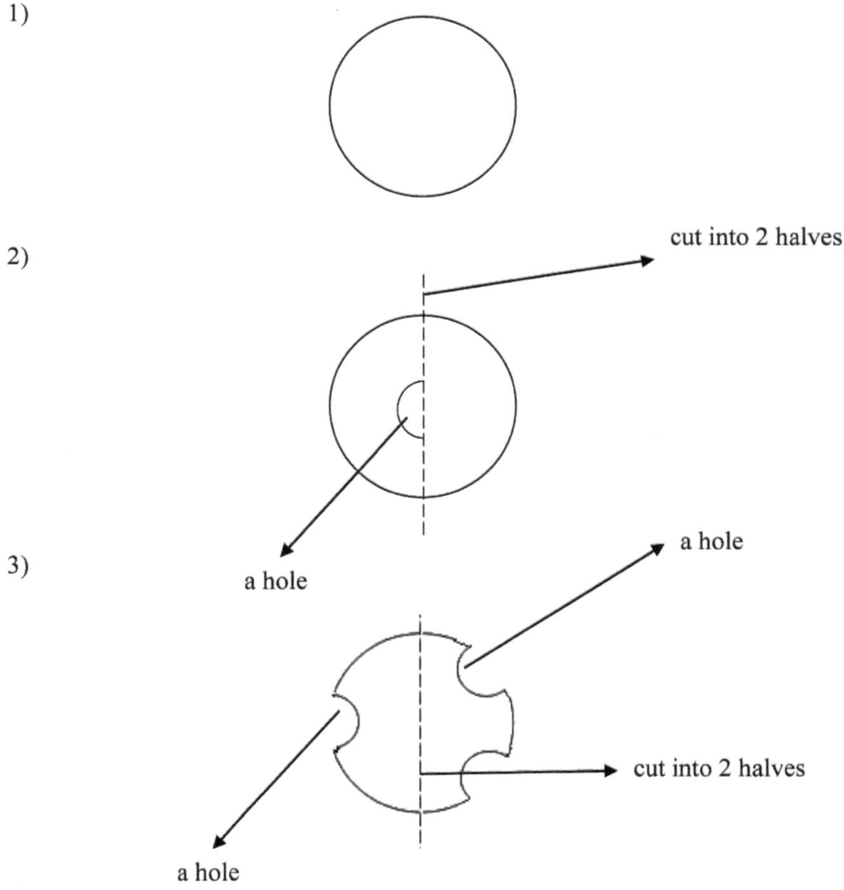

Figure 33B. The ping-pong balls – parts of the sentence

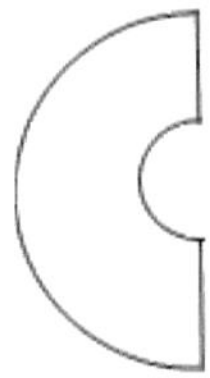	SUBJECT
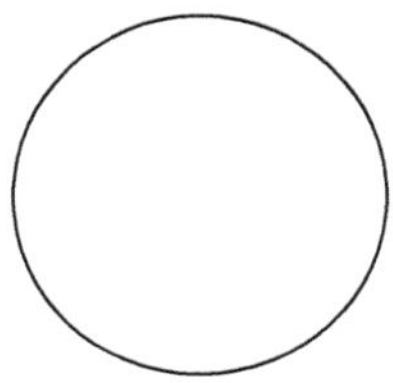	PREDICATE
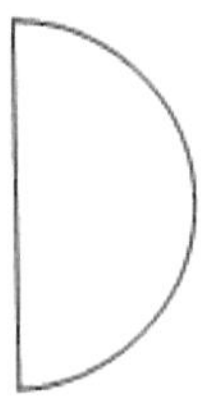	OBJECT
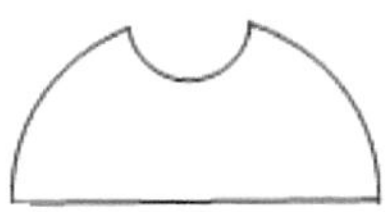	AUXILIARY VERB
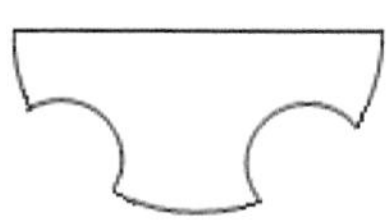	AUXILIARY VERB (NEGATIVE)

Figure 33C. The ping-pong sentence structure; types of sentences

1. affirmative statement

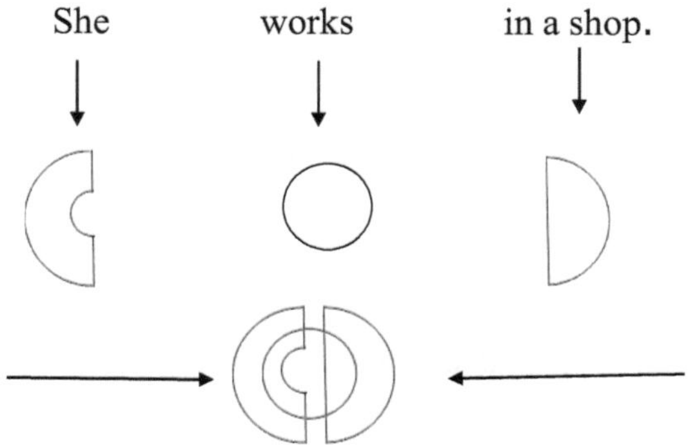

2. negative statement

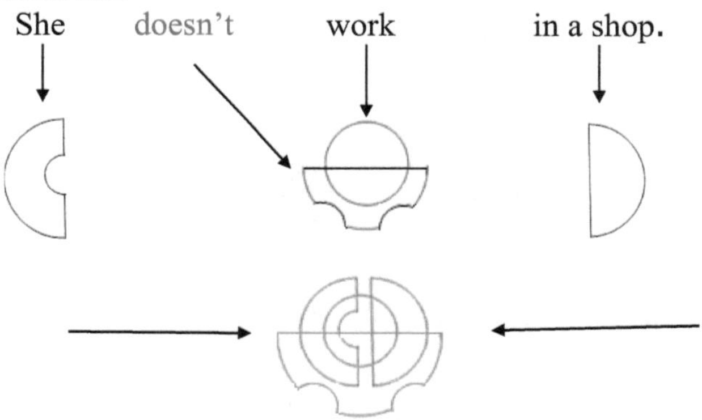

3. question

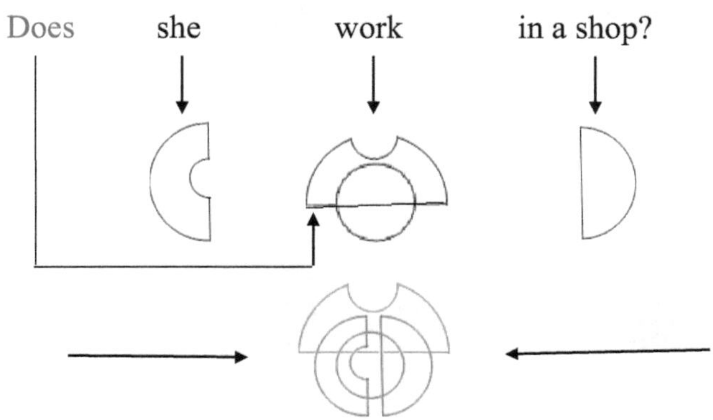

➢ **The magnetic sentence system**

The magnetic sentence system is used to develop the correct usage of grammar structures through the haptic and audible involvement of a set of magnetic balls and sticks, called the "magnetix". Each word goes in parallel with one magnetic element (Figure 34); one element is fixed to another, forming a chain sentence. Longer structures create shapes of buildings that could be utilised in a word-named shape, thus practising lexis. During the forming process of the magnetix, students repeat words loudly. After the final element-word occurs, a person revises a whole sentence. The variety of possibilities offered by the magnetic system structure influences the effectiveness and consistency of grammar and lexical layers, acquired through the auditory-tactile channel.

Figure 34. The magnetic sentence system – grammar chain structure

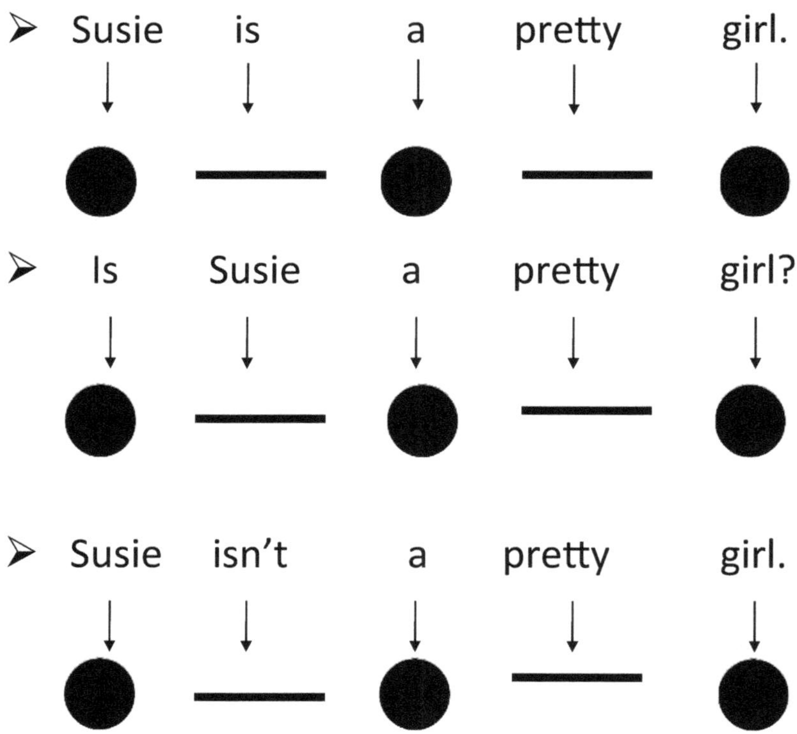

➢ **Tactile knots sentences**

The sentence, in this association, has been compared to a rope or a washing line covered with bumps – i.e., words that make the sentence plateau lumpy.

Students compose a sentence by connecting separate words – knots, on a washing line or string – in one joined structure (Figure 35). During loud repetition of words, the visually handicapped tie knots on the string. One knot transforms into one word.

Students who make grammar or pronunciation mistakes are obliged to tie an extra knot; one mistake equals one extra knot. It is worth noticing that diverse types of string were related to different grammar structures.

Tactile knot sentences were recognised as a productive teaching aid, albeit one with a bizarre form of implementation in the language learning-teaching process, but structurally effective nonetheless.

Figure 35. The tactile repetition of grammar structures – "tactile knots"

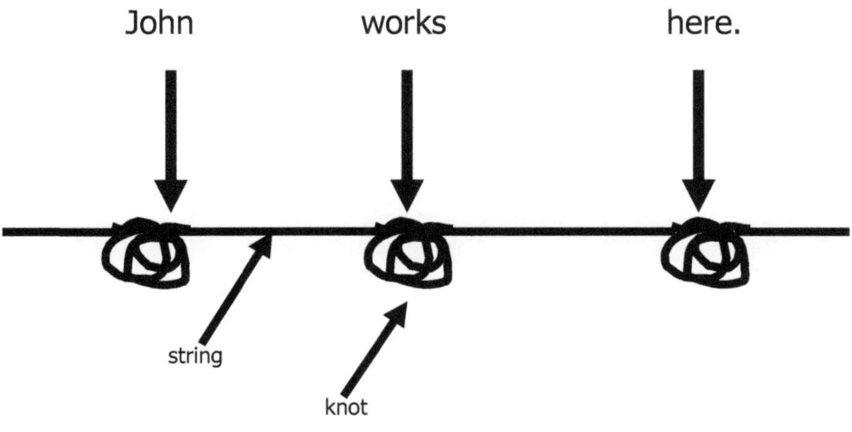

5.8. Classroom design

One of the areas among my considerations was class arrangement. Designing a classroom appears to be as crucial as the method itself. The creation of the proper physical arrangements supports the process of achieving a communicative level of English (Hadfield, 2002).

To reach the goals of the therapy, students sat comfortably within the round-shaped learning-teaching environment, with the teacher standing in the middle of the circle (Figure 36A). The circle-shaped environment was designed to make students clearly audible. The focus was placed on proper audibility, due to the students' hearing disorders that accompany the visual impairment. Two of them were recognised as partly deaf-blind, being only right-ear listeners.

Figure 36A. The Re-charged Direct Method classroom management

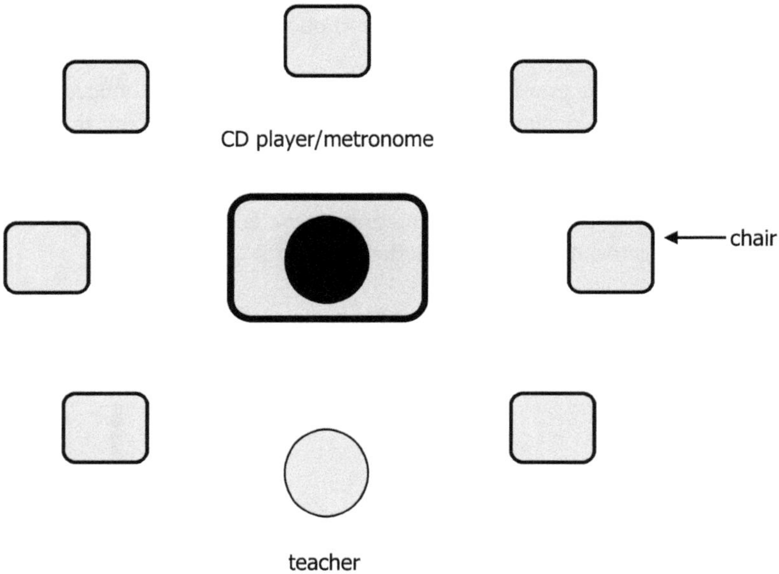

Water or collage clusters were rectangular-shaped arrangements; students were seated at a table, having bowls filled with water or sandtrays in front of them (Figure 36B).

Figure 36B. The water/collage classroom design

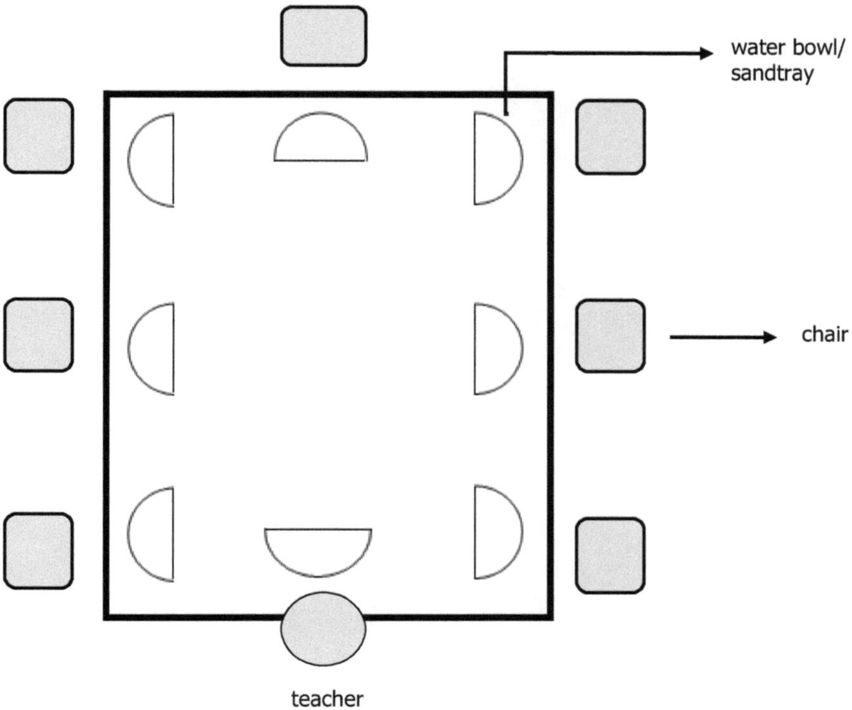

Chapter Six: Research

6.0. Introductory remarks

Chapter 5 discusses the format of the research and states the research problem and hypotheses. The chapter outlines the content and composition of the training tools, and focuses on areas directly pertinent to the research aims. It also provides information on the research methodology and subjects, the evaluation and scoring systems used to analyse the intensity of positive and negative emotions within the Positive and Negative Affect Schedule (PANAS questionnaire), placement, and achievement tests in L2. The chapter concludes with an outline of the research, including both qualitative and quantitative results gained in the PLT study.

6.1. The purpose of the research

The purpose of my research was to create a psycho-linguistic therapy that is not simply a conversation, but a therapy that has form and substance, created on the basis of my theoretical orientation, and – what seems to be crucial – a therapy that embodies language input, showing practicum in relation to the interaction between visually impaired students and the English teacher. The psycho-linguistic therapy "Touching the World" has not yet been the focus of any research involving the correlation between positive and negative affects and language acquisition. Essentially, my dissertation endeavours to investigate the intensity of emotions during the teaching-learning process. It is expected that the challenges created during the PLT induce mental balance within linguistic development.

It seemed to me vital to propose a study that would aim at exploring language as a therapy tool seen through the intensity of activation.

The **thesis** of the present study is *"Teaching English as a foreign language to the visually impaired students"*.

The **research problem** I found worth solving corresponds with the question:

Is teaching English as a foreign language to visually impaired students within the psycho-linguistic therapy "Touching the World" a tool that influences achievements in L2 and the intensity of affects?

I hope that my findings will be useful to teachers of English working with visually impaired adult students.

6.2. Description of the sample

The psycho-linguistic therapy "Touching the World" was set up in the school years 2004/2005 with group 1 (an experimental group), and in 2005/2006 with two groups working in parallel, one experimental (group 2) and a control group (group 3). The therapy covered 10 months from September till June, two sessions per week, 6 or 8 sessions per month, 74 sessions per year (Table 1).

Table 1. The PLT timetable

Month	Number of weeks	Frequency in a week	Number of sessions
September	4	2	8
October	4	2	8
November	4	2	8
December	3	2	6
January	4	2	8
February	4	2	8
March	4	2	8
April	3	2	6
May	4	2	8
June	3	2	6
total	**37**	**2**	**74**

The study was carried out on a population of 23 learners, 15 females and 8 males. The subjects involved in the research were visually impaired Polish adults. The age of participants ranged from 19 to 55 and the mean age of the sample was 33.6 years (SD=11.4). Participants were recruited from the Polish Association for the Blind in Bialystok, Poland. The mean number of English language education (years) was 4.34 (SD=1.19), with a range of 0–10 years of linguistic experience, and the mean number of visual impairment (years) was 18.2 (SD=16.4): 7 people blind since birth, and 16 people with visual impairment acquired later in their lives.

Descriptions of the groups

Age – 19–55 years old
Disability – visual impairment, partly deaf-blind

Level of English (language competence) – absolute beginners, false beginners, and experienced beginners. The constant problem that appeared was their low level of linguistic competences in Polish.

Group 1

Disability – 3 blind students, 4 visually impaired
Number of students – 7

- 2 students with no English learning experience
- 1 student with 3-year experience with learning English
- 2 students with 4-year experience with learning English
- 2 students with 7-year experience with learning English

Group 2

Disability – 2 blind students, 6 visually impaired
Number of students – 8

- 4 students with no English learning experience
- 1 student with 3-year experience with learning English
- 2 students with 5-year experience with learning English
- 1 student with 7-year experience with learning English

Group 3

Disability – 3 blind students, 5 visually impaired
Number of students – 8

- 2 students with no English learning experience
- 3 students with 3-year experience with learning English
- 2 students with 4-year experience with learning English
- 1 student with 7-year experience with learning English

Level of education/achieved qualifications – secondary school, 1 diploma in economics, unemployed, living on a pension or lacking any professional activity.

The number of students during the PLT study was based on representativeness, which is the most common practice in quantitative studies. According to the Polish Association for the Blind, there were 376 visually impaired people in Bialystok, from the ages of 16–60, in 2004 and 2005, and 372 in 2006. The minimal value of the sample for the PANAS questionnaire was 11 subjects, d=5 points (d equals minimal numerical sample), while the PLT groups consisted of 15 students; for the achievement tests in L2 the minimal value was equal to

8 subjects, d=2 points, while the group itself consisted of 15 subjects. This indicates that the number of students in the PLT groups was sufficient to consider groups 1 and 2 representative for the research.

The success of PLT group cooperation was focused on different issues:

- They had a sense of direction as the PLT group.
- There was positive, supportive atmosphere, members felt secure enough to express their individualities.
- They were able to work together productively.
- They were open-minded, flexible, and receptive to new ideas.

6.3. Research hypotheses

The aim of the thesis was to solve the research problem: "Is teaching English to visually impaired students within the PLT a therapeutic tool influencing the intensity of positive and negative affects?" This was pursued by verifying three research hypotheses:

Hypothesis 1

The psycho-linguistic therapy "Touching the World" influences positive affects. The first research hypothesis formulated for the purpose of the present study examines the claim that the psycho-linguistic therapy "Touching the World" influences the increase in the intensity of positive affects.

Hypothesis 2

The psycho-linguistic therapy "Touching the World" influences negative affects. The hypothesis explores the impacts of the psycho-linguistic therapy "Touching the World" on a decrease in the intensity of negative affects.

Hypothesis 3

The psycho-linguistic therapy "Touching the World" influences language communicative competences.
According to the third research hypothesis the visually impaired students develop linguistic competences within the psycho-linguistic therapy "Touching the World".

6.4. Methodology

For the purpose of this dissertation qualitative and quantitative research was carried out. The qualitative approach allows not only to find the root of the research problem but also to examine the relationship between variables. There are two kinds of variables identified in the research – independent and dependent (Rugg and Petre, 2007):

(1) *Independent variable:*
   - visual impairment.

(2) *Dependent variables:*
   - the intensity of positive affects,
   - the intensity of negative affects,
   - achievements in L2.

Various types of case study involved in my research offered insight into the issue of the PLT and allowed generalisations to be made referring to the background theory. Stake (2000) enumerates three types of case study research that appear in my thesis: intrinsic, instrumental and collective. The intrinsic case study is applied when a researcher wants a detailed understanding of the particular case. During the instrumental case study the researcher wants to understand the phenomenon through an analysis of a case to provide an insight into an issue or to redraw a generalisation. The last type of case study format refers to the collective case study, where a researcher "investigates numerous cases to study a phenomenon, group, condition, or event" (Stake, 2000:445).

For my dissertation it was possible and practical to apply both strategies: the inductive one to develop the theory and the deductive strategy to test the constructed theory using data gathered from the set of cases with a reliance on current theory.

6.4.1. Triangulation

To obtain construct validity I strove for triangulation, defined as "a combination of methods used to study the interrelated phenomena from multiple and different angles or perspectives" (Bogdan and Biklen, 2006:101).

The PLT research was designed to be a triangulation of data resources and time involvement:

- Triangulation of data sources – I drew evidence from a variety of data sources trying to verify the same set of findings. Each student was the source of data, so participant triangulation focused on gathering information from 23 subjects: the same affective traits were seen from different individual perspectives.
- Time triangulation – collecting data from various periods of time. The PANAS questionnaire was repeated four times, every three months. Achievement tests were given three times per year (Table 2).

Table 2. The PLT evaluations

Month	Number of evaluations	Type of evaluations	
September	2	PANAS	L_2
December	1	PANAS	-
January	1	-	L_2
March	1	PANAS	-
June	2	PANAS	L_2

With regard to internal validity I took the following steps:

- data in each case study were analysed using the earlier described pattern matching approach for dependent variables, whereby each hypothesis contained a single, measurable dependent variable,
- to increase contrast between solutions only two dichotomous patterns were used: an increase in positive affects or decrease in negative emotions were measured by two variables, the third variable measured the achievement in L2 of the visually impaired students.

In my thesis I used various sources of evidence to establish convergent lines of inquiry in the process of triangulation to confirm the findings.

6.5. Instruments

Three major sources of data are included in the research:

(1) **a PANAS questionnaire** (Appendix A),
(2) **a placement test** (Appendix D),
(3) **achievement tests** (Appendices E and F).

I administered the **PANAS questionnaire** with time-frames ranging from "right now" to "during last year". PANAS evaluation was taken four times a year: every three months: in September, then December, March, and June to confirm its reliability of the intensity of affects changes within the groups. The test was administered one-on-one at a time. Respondents were asked to rate orally (after my reading and translation) the extent to which they experienced each particular emotion within a specified time period with reference to a 5-point Likert scale. The questionnaire took 10 minutes per student.

Scoring instructions (Watson et al., 1988):

Positive Affect Score:
The score covered the sum of 10 positive items: 1, 3, 5, 9, 10, 12, 14, 16, 17, 19. A higher score indicates a more positive affect, or the extent to which the individual feels enthusiastic, active, and alert. The numbers are related to definite positive affects: 1.interested, 3.excited, 5.strong, 9.enthusiastic, 10.proud, 12.alert, 14.inspired, 16.determined, 17.attentive, 19.active.

Scores can range from the minimum number of 10 points to the maximum of 50; higher scores represent higher levels of positive affect.

Negative Affect Score:
The score was calculated within 10 negative items: 2, 4, 6, 7, 8, 11, 13, 15, 18, 20. A higher score indicates a more negative affect, or the extent to which the individual feels aversive mood states and general distress. The numbers are related to definite negative affects: 2.distress, 4.upset, 6.guilty, 7.scared, 8.hostile, 11.irritable, 13.ashamed, 15.nervous, 18.jiterry, 20.afraid.

Scores can range from the minimum number of 10 points to maximum 50, with lower scores representing lower levels of negative affect.

In cases with internally missing data (items not answered), the sums were computed after imputation of the missing values: items on scale/actually answered, multiplied by the sum obtained from the answered items.

I designed a placement test and achievement tests in L2 to determine the students' degree of language skills for the purpose of placing them in the efficient linguistic process during the psycho-linguistic therapy "Touching the World".

The placement test consists of 30 open questions; scores range from 0 to 30; 1 point per question. It takes 15 minutes.

Achievement tests in L2 include:

5 multiple choice questions, 5 open questions, 5 ping-pong sentence structures to build, 5 water sentences created within the grammar water jar technique, 5 dicto-listening sentences put into a sandtray building task, 5 mistaken statements within the tactile knots technique.

The test lasts 45 minutes; scores range from 0 to 30, 1 point per answer.

6.6. Data collection and analysis

The research presents achievements in L2 and the effects of the independent variable (visual impairment) on dependent variables (the intensity of positive and negative affects) without ambiguity.

The techniques of data collection included observations, questionnaires and critical self-reflection. Applied triangulation enabled me to enhance data verification.

Data collection was considered on two-layered involvement: mental, measuring emotions, divided into two modules of positive and negative affects covered by PANAS questionnaires; and linguistic, focused on achievement tests in L2.

To link the data and find out which hypotheses were true, I used the pattern matching approach which is a well-documented analysis technique in case study. The basic idea here was to describe two patterns – one closely fitting the research hypotheses and an alternative one constituting a rival explanation. Then the research data were compared with both patterns to see which explanation matches the data better. It is worth noting that when using pattern matching emphasises, every hypothesis contains a pair of variables (independent and dependent) which are proposed to be linked in some kind of relationship (Rugg and Petre, 2007). To build an adequate explanation and present these insights in a convincing manner I used the following measures:

- every hypothesis was verified on the basis of measurable variables denoting specific changes in emotions,
- it was checked if literal replication occurred, which in my research was about finding out if the intensity of affects within the continuum shows similar changes in emotional development,
- it was checked if theoretical replication took place, if my prediction that higher levels of positive, emotional development occur in parallel with the development of language acquisition,
- simple statistical techniques were used to provide objective confirmation of relationships: it must be stressed that this was not an attempt at formulating statistical generalisations, but merely to obtain clear and subjective interpretation criteria.

The whole process of analysis, which is typical and advisable for the case study method, started not only after all data from every case were collected, but just after the first observations. Making use of flexibility of methods and methodological triangulation, I conducted the basic analysis after gathering data from each source and during data gathering.

I monitored all the irrelevant variables in order to see whether the independent variable actually affects the dependent variable. The observation of behaviour of the visually impaired students during the PLT did not involve manipulation of an independent variable with certainty. The same instruments and variables – independent and dependent – were indicators of measurement of positive and negative affects and achievements in L2 in three groups.

For the sake of simplicity, the findings of the research are described in accordance with the subsequent research hypotheses. In each of them, the presentation of descriptive statistics is followed by statistical findings.

Following the deductive strategy, my main objective in the study was to solve the research problem by verifying a set of three hypotheses. Four PANAS questionnaires were administered to the students to verify hypotheses 1 and 2.

Research hypothesis 1: The PLT influences positive affects.
Independent variable: visual impairment
Dependent variable: the intensity of positive affects

GROUP 1
Questionnaire 1 (September, 2004) shows the initial mean scores of positive affects at the beginning of the PLT that range from 1.28 to 1.71. The lowest scores correlate with being inspired: 1.28 and excited: 1.29. The scores in the mid position focus on active: 1.43, proud: 1.57, enthusiastic: 1.71 and interested: 1.71. The highest mean scores appear in relation to alert and attentive, having the same mean value of 4.43. It is worth noticing that 7 affects are the lowest with the modes ranging from 1.0 and 2.0; an emphasis is put on the intensity of very slightly or a little on a 5-point Likert scale that confirms a very low positive affect of the visually impaired students at the beginning of the PLT.

In **questionnaire 2** (December, 2004) the highest score indicates the intensity of being alert: 4.29, with the similar mean score, appearing in questionnaire 1, probably (as the students emphasised) due to their visual impairment, that corresponds with being permanently watchful. The mode circulates around 2.57 for interested, enthusiastic and determined suggesting higher rates of the intensity than presented in questionnaire 1, with the modes equalling 2–3 for 8 trait scores. The lowest scores appear in connection with proud: 1.86 and active: 2.00 with a tendency to increase.

Questionnaire 3 (March, 2005) correlates with modes for 1 score between 4 and 5, 5 scores for 3–4, and 4 scores focused on 2–3 modes. The highest scores cover such traits like alert: 4.29 on the same level in questionnaire 2, attentive: 3.86, interested: 3.57 and enthusiastic: 3.43, with 1-point difference between questionnaires 2 and 3. The lowest scores vary from 2.29 for proud to 2.86 for determined. The increase in modes and mean scores underlines changes of positive affects during the PLT, observed in research 1.

Questionnaire 4 (June, 2005) indicates means of the highest scores for 4 traits: interested, enthusiastic, alert, inspired from 4.14. to 4.29 with 4–5-point modes. 5 scores are around modes 3–4, from 3.14 to 3.71 for excited, strong, determined, attentive and active. It emphasises that the number of rising scores is permanently increasing. The lowest position occupies just one trait – proud: 2.57, within the mode that ranges between 2–3.

Table 3. Mean scores of positive affects – group 1

Positive Affects - group 1										
	interested	excited	strong	enthusiastic	proud	alert	inspired	determined	attentive	active
questionnaire 1	1.71	1.29	2.00	1.71	1.57	4.43	1.28	1.86	4.43	1.43
questionnaire 2	2.57	2.14	2.43	2.57	1.86	4.29	2.43	2.57	2.29	2.00
questionnaire 3	3.57	3.00	2.71	3.43	2.29	4.29	3.29	2.86	3.86	2.71
questionnaire 4	4.14	3.57	3.14	4.29	2.57	4.14	4.14	3.43	3.71	3.57

Figure 37 demonstrates the increase in all affect traits except alert and attentive, seen as an impediment of visual impairment that the students share. The highest levels of positive values cover enthusiastic, interested and inspired. The decrease of alert and attentive can be considered as progressively positive due to its connection with relaxation techniques within the PLT that helped release the physically and mentally conditioned tension they feel.

Figure 37. Positive affect changes – group 1

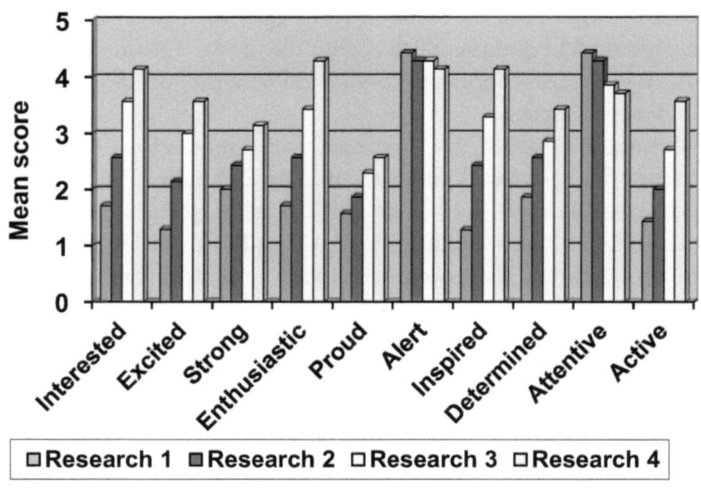

Table 4 indicates the change of the intensity of positive affects (Oleś, 1992) between research 1 and research 4. The initial value corresponds with 17.3 but the final research: 32.6 correlates within a double value increase. The dimension of change between research 1 and 4 equals 15.3. The highest rate of increase appears between research 1 and 2 and covers 5.6; the comparison between research 2 and 3 indicates the rate of change on 4.8 level, whereas research 3 and 4 are almost on the same intensity rate equal 4.9.

Table 4. The level of the intensity of positive affects – group 1

Intensity of positive affects			
R 1	R 2	R 3	R 4
17.3	22.9	27.7	32.6

R1 – Research 1

GROUP 2

Questionnaire 1 (September, 2005) presents 7 initial means on the level of 1–2 mode scale, with a range of the lowest scores – proud: 1.25, excited: 1.38, and the mid scores oscillate between 1.50 for enthusiastic and active and 2.00 for determined. The highest values are represented by attentive: 3.75 and alert: 3.88. In comparison with group 1, the same traits occupy the highest positions: alert and attentive. Affects of being interested and strong indicate the same mean score.

Questionnaire 2 (December, 2005) involves 6 means that are developed on the rate of 6 traits around the mode of 2–3, that form the lowest values. 3 scores associated with inspired: 3.00, enthusiastic: 3.13 and attentive: 3.63 are located between 3–4 on a Likert scale and one – alert occupies the rate just above 4. Similarly to questionnaire 1, alert and attentive reach the highest scores.

Questionnaire 3 (March, 2006) compared with questionnaire 2 indicates 8 mean scores: on a very high level of intensity, between 3–4 on the scale. The highest position is reached by inspired: 4.00, enthusiastic: 3.88, attentive: 3.75, interested and determined with 3.63. 2 means are seen as the lowest ones indicating the values for strong: 2.38 and proud with 2.88.

Questionnaire 4 (June, 2006) correlates with 6 traits of very high mode position: 4–5 that means quite a bit and extremely. The highest level – 4.50, employs enthusiastic and inspired, then interested: 4.25, determined and attentive with 4.13. The lowest means shape around 2.88 for strong, with an emphasis put on physical and mental meanings; the same score – 3.19 is seen for excited and active.

Table 5. Mean scores of positive affects – group 2

Positive Affects – group 2										
	interested	excited	strong	enthusiastic	proud	alert	inspired	determined	attentive	active
questionnaire 1	1.63	1.38	1.63	1.50	1.25	3.88	1.75	2.00	3.75	1.50
questionnaire 2	2.88	2.88	2.25	3.13	2.38	4.13	3.00	2.88	3.63	2.88
questionnaire 3	3.63	3.50	2.38	3.88	2.88	3.88	4.00	3.63	3.75	3.25
questionnaire 4	4.25	3.75	2.88	4.50	3.63	4.00	4.50	4.13	4.13	3.75

Figure 38 presents the positive affect change, related to the traits – inspired, enthusiastic, and interested – that reach the highest levels. All affects are in progress, except for alert that fluctuates on the constant level. The lowest trait corresponds with strong; the students find the affect as physically and mentally conditioned with an emphasis put on their disability that blocks strength.

Figure 38. Positive affect changes – group 2

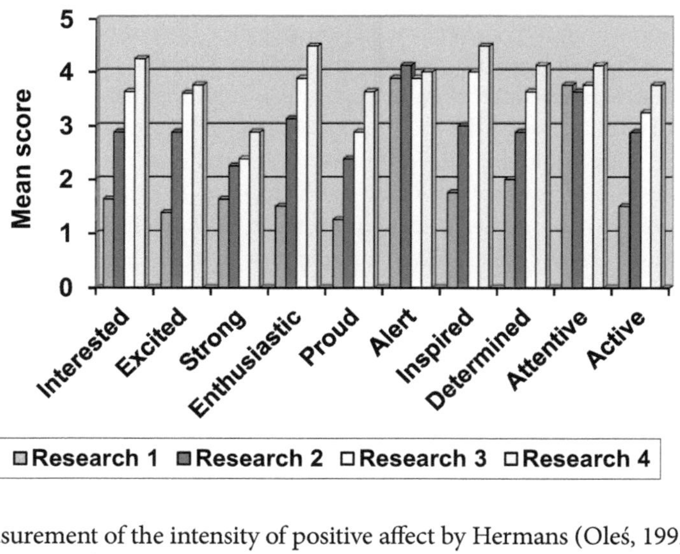

The measurement of the intensity of positive affect by Hermans (Oleś, 1992) evaluates the rates of saturation that indicate quantitative changes between research 1:16.4 and 4:35.5. (Table 6). The rate of change equals 19.1 and is 3.8 higher than in group 1. The highest difference refers to research 1 and 2 with the result of 9.5. Research 2 and 3 focus on 5.00. The lowest number of change correlates with research 3 and 4, achieving the position of 4.6. Such comparison indicates the highest intensity change of positive affect between research 1 and 2.

Table 6. The level of the intensity of positive affects – group 2

Intensity of positive affects			
R 1	R 2	R 3	R 4
16.4	25.9	30.9	35.5

R1 – Research 1

GROUP 3 (control group)

Questionnaire 1 (September, 2005) employs the highest results within the traits – alert: 3.75 and attentive: 3.63, emphasising the independent variable – visual impairment shared in three research groups. The lowest levels evolve on enthusiastic: 1.38, strong and active: 1.50.

6 results fluctuate within modes 2–3.

Questionnaire 2 (December, 2005) focuses on a noticeable decrease in alert: 3.75:1.75, determined: 2.13:1.63, attentive: 3.63:2.00, and an increase in interested, excited and strong. 4 scores oscillate within 2.00: excited, strong, enthusiastic and attentive. 4 results: determined, active with the score of 1.63, proud, alert: 1.73 are located below 2.00, two left – interested: 2.25 and inspired: 2.38 are above 2.00.

In **questionnaire 3** (March, 2006) the mean values are formed around 2.00 and a bit above. The clear difference between group 1 and 2 is seen in tendency for decrease in positive affects or just appearing on the similar level. The decline in traits is represented by interested: 2.25:2.13, inspired: 2.38:2.00; excited stays on the constant level of 2.00. The rise in the results is changing within the minimal value ranging from 0.12 to 0.38.

Questionnaire 4 (June, 2006) corresponds with a decrease in indicators of 4 traits – proud: 2.00:1.75, inspired: 2.00:1.88, attentive: 2.25:1.63, active: 1.75:1.63. The same progress level, not changed, is covered in questionnaire 3, and represented by interested: 2.13, alert: 1.88, determined: 2.00. Positive emotional development circulates around modules – excited: 2.13, strong: 2.25 and enthusiastic: 2.38. It is worth noticing that the mode is focused on rates between 1 and 2.50.

Table 7. Mean scores of positive affects – group 3

Positive Affects - group 3										
	interested	excited	strong	enthusiastic	proud	alert	inspired	determined	attentive	active
questionnaire 1	2.00	1.88	1.50	1.38	1.63	3.75	1.75	2.13	3.63	1.50
questionnaire 2	2.25	2.00	2.00	2.00	1.75	1.75	2.38	1.63	2.00	1.63
questionnaire 3	2.13	2.00	2.13	2.25	2.00	1.88	2.00	2.00	2.25	1.75
questionnaire 4	2.13	2.13	2.25	2.38	1.75	1.88	1.88	2.00	1.63	1.63

The figure below indicates fluctuations of interested, proud, inspired, determined and active with no clear indicator of positive affect change. The minimal progress is seen in the following modules: interested, excited. Inspired and active share the pattern of decline. The mean scores circulate around 2.00, besides alert and attentive that suggest a huge incomprehensible, accidental decline in comparison with groups 1 and 2.

Figure 39. Positive affect changes – group 3

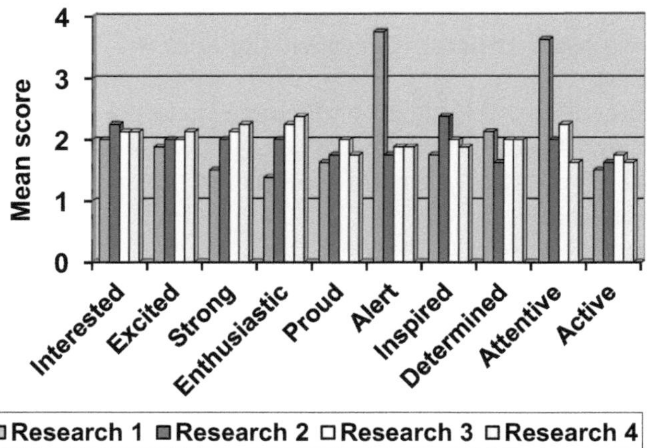

The indicator of positive affect (Oleś, 1992) confirms the rates of fluctuations of the mean scores with the tendency, firstly to decline, and then increase about 0.4, emphasising the constant process but not progressive (Table 8).

Table 8. The level of the intensity of positive affects – group 3

Intensity of positive affects			
R 1	R 2	R 3	R 4
17.4	17.3	18.5	17.8

R1 – Research 1

According to Whiskers' plot, two groups of traits are seen in research 1 – for groups 1,2,3 (Figure 40):

- the first set: alert and attentive circulates within standard deviations of 3.0–5.0;
- the second set: interested, excited, strong, enthusiastic, proud, inspired, determined and active with standard deviations fluctuating from 0.8 to 2.7. The trait of being determined covers the highest standard deviation score.

Figure 40. The Box and Whiskers plot for positive affects – research 1

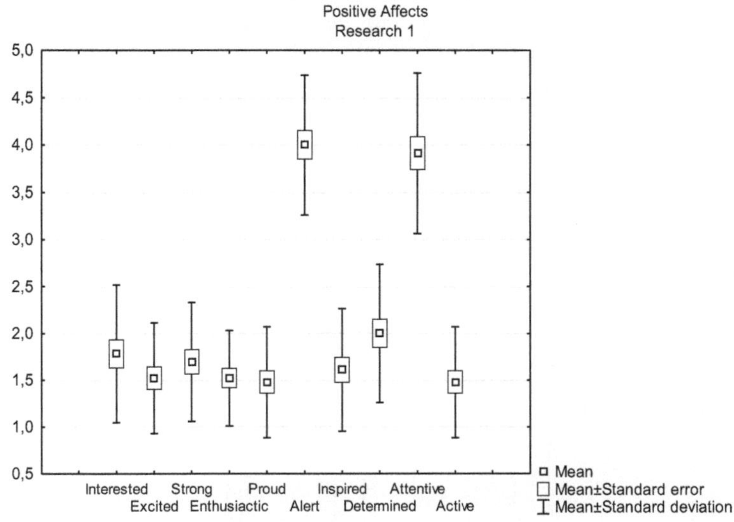

Research 2 (Figure 41) indicates the initial value of the scale, different from research 1, beginning with 1.0 (R1=0.5). The flattening of the scale is noticeable. The highest standard deviations cover the values of 2.0–5.0, one point lower than it was pointed in research 1. The differentiation between two groups of traits does not exist in the box plot.

Figure 41. The Box and Whiskers plot for positive affects – research 2

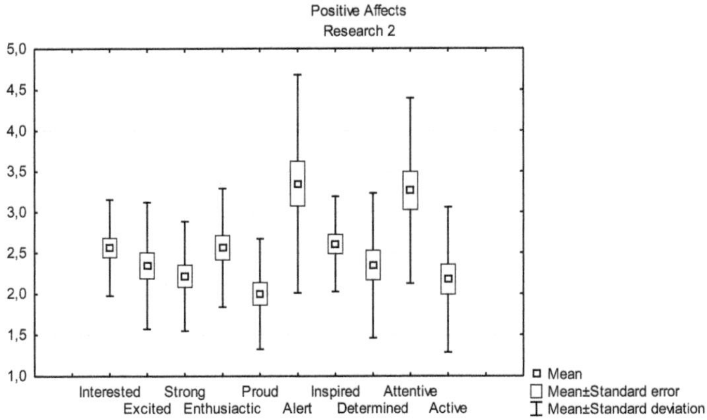

The box plot related to research 3 (Figure 42) describes the mid position of affects, with standard deviations scores grouped between 1.5–4.5. The lower boundaries (strong and proud) of the intensity of positive affect rise systematically. The highest positions are occupied by alert and attentive. Interested, enthusiastic and inspired are related to the average standard deviation that circulates around 3.0.

Figure 42. The Box and Whiskers plot for positive affects – research 3

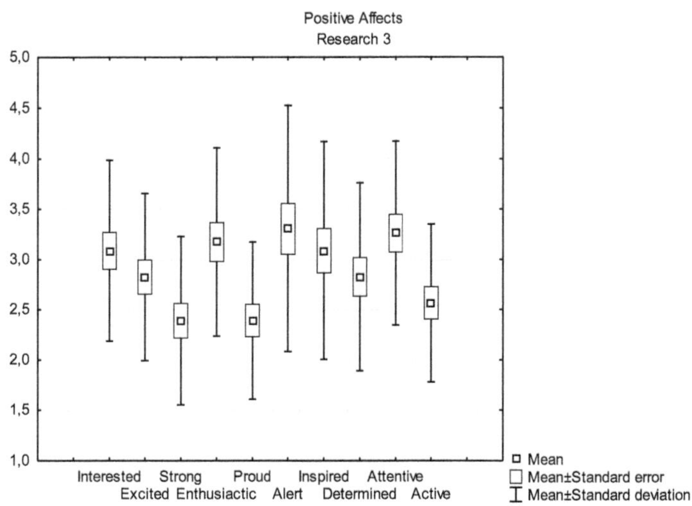

Research 4 (Figure 43) presents traits grouped around 3.0–4.0; only three traits are located below 3.0: strong, proud and active on the lowest edge of 1.6. In comparison with research 1, most traits were between 1.0–2.5 except alert and attentive; it suggests about 1.5 change of the intensity of positive affects. The highest level is covered by enthusiastic, inspired and interested. The box plot correlates with the average standard deviation, fluctuating between 2.0–4.5.

Figure 43. The Box and Whiskers plot for positive affects – research 4

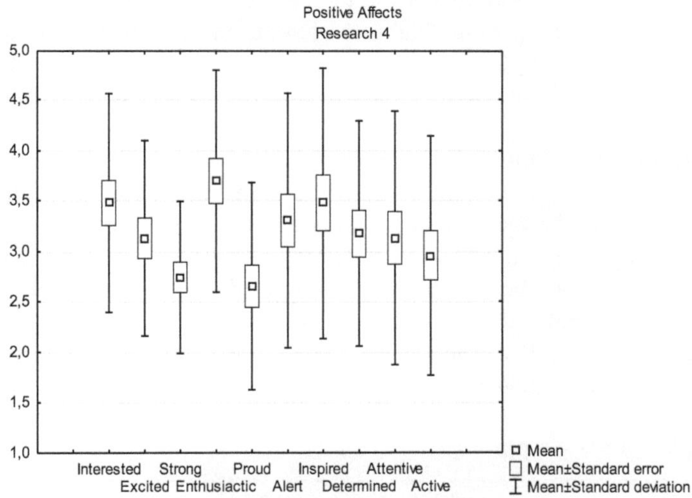

Research hypothesis 2: The PLT influences negative affects.
Independent variable: visual impairment
Dependent variable: the intensity of negative affects

GROUP 1

Questionnaire 1 (September, 2004) correlates with the highest intensity zone of mean scores, being around 4.00: afraid, nervous and irritable: 4.29. The mid values are occupied by distressed: 3.85 and scared: 3.71. The lowest level is represented by hostile: 1.43, guilty: 2.00, and jittery: 2.43. The mean scores circulate from 1.43 to 4.29. The mode positions are located around 3.00–4.00. The students explained the intensity of negative affects, underlining the environment of visual impairment they shared. The feeling of physical and mental fear is closely related to this dysfunction.

Questionnaire 2 (December, 2004) in comparison with 1, incorporates the highest means of 4.00 for irritable, 3.57 for distressed and afraid. The lowest scores appear in relation to hostile: 1.14, jittery: 1.57 and guilty: 1.71. The average values are represented by nervous: 3.00, scared: 3.29 and upset: 2.29. The mode is seen around 3.5; it indicates a decreasing tendency for the intensity of negative activation.

Data in **questionnaire 3** (March, 2005) circulates around 1 – on a Likert scale. Five scores cover 1.00–2.00 – hostile: 1.14, jittery: 1.29, ashamed: 1.43, upset and guilty: 1.71. The level of achieved values indicates a decreasing tendency of negative affects. The highest position is absorbed by afraid: 3.00, distressed: 2.86. The mode appears around 1.00. The average scores fluctuate around 2.57 for irritable and nervous: 2.71. The mode difference between research 2 and 3 covers a 2.5 decrease.

Questionnaire 4 (June, 2005) presents 7 mean scores on the lowest level around 1.00 – jittery and hostile: 1.00, nervous, ashamed and upset: 1.14, guilty: 1.29, scared: 1.43. The measured median is 1.5. The mode value is 1.00. Three scores are formed around 2.00 – irritable: 2.00, distressed: 2.29 and afraid: 2.57. The number of 7 scores below 2.00 emphasises the decrease of means in connection with questionnaire 1. The highest indicators are located around 2.00–3.00. The lowest values oscillate around 1.00–2.00. In questionnaire 1 just one trait is grouped around 1.00–2.00, in questionnaire 4 more than 50%.

Table 9. Mean scores of negative affects – group 1

Negative Affects - group 1										
	distressed	**upset**	**guilty**	**scared**	**hostile**	**irritable**	**ashamed**	**nervous**	**jittery**	**afraid**
questionnaire 1	3.85	2.86	2.00	3.71	1.43	4.29	2.71	4.00	2.43	4.00
questionnaire 2	3.57	2.71	1.71	3.29	1.14	4.00	2.29	3.00	1.57	3.57
questionnaire 3	2.86	1.71	1.71	2.71	1.14	2.57	1.43	2.71	1.29	3.00
questionnaire 4	2.29	1.14	1.29	1.43	1.00	2.00	1.14	1.14	1.00	2.57

Figure 44 presents a change of the intensity of negative affects. The decrease in negative activation is seen through the fluctuations of all traits. The highest values: 4.00–4.50, are achieved by irritable, nervous and afraid. The lowest position is covered by guilty: 2.00. Comparing research 1 with research 4, the highest difference exists between the means of irritable, scared, nervous and jittery on

50% level, noticeably lower in research 1 than in research 4. The lowest difference occupies guilty and hostile.

Figure 44. Negative affect changes – group 1

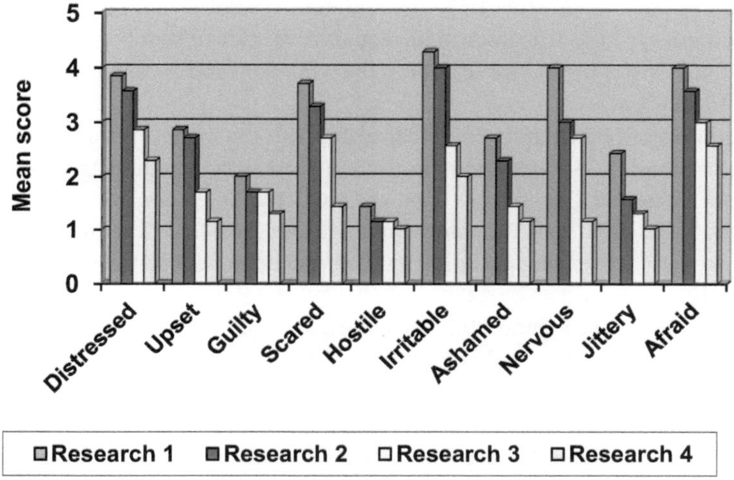

Herman's indicator of negative affects (Oleś, 1992) between research 1 and 4 is correlated around 50% decrease: 16.3. The highest dimension is achieved between research 3 and 4 – 6.1. The lowest difference appears between research 1 and 2 and equals 4.4. (Table 10).

Table 10. The level of the intensity of negative affects – group 1

Intensity of negative affects			
R 1	R 2	R 3	R 4
31.3	26.9	21.1	15.0

R1 – Research 1

GROUP 2

In **questionnaire 1** (September, 2005) the highest mean scores of negative activation are concentrated around 4.00 – distressed: 4.00, upset: 4.00 and scared: 4.13. The mid position values are occupied with irritable, nervous, afraid: 3.88 and jittery: 3.63. The lowest level is presented by guilty and hostile: 1.75. The mode covers 3.6. 50% of scores are located between 3.00–4.00; 3 values appear between 4.00–5.00, underlining the high intensity of negative activation.

Questionnaire 2 (December, 2005) depicts a decreasing tendency for all negative affects. The highest difference equals 1.50 and is visible in relation to upset, nervous: 1.25, 1.13: scared, 1.00: irritable and jittery. The highest zone is seen through distressed: 3.38, scared and afraid: 3.00. The lowest scores are represented by guilty and hostile: 1.63. The midlevel correlates with upset: 2.50, nervous and jittery: 2.63. The mode value equals 2.00. 50% of scores appear between 2.00–3.00. Only 3 means are seen between 3.00–4.00 and 2 are found within the area of 1.00–2.00.

Questionnaire 3 (March, 2006) correlates with the highest rates of distressed: 3.00 and afraid: 2.38; both affects indicate a decreasing tendency in comparison with questionnaire 2 that equals 0.38. and 0.62. The lowest level is covered by jittery and guilty: 1.50 with the values ranging from 1.13–0.13. The mid area of the mean scores is represented by upset, irritable and nervous: 1.88 with about 1-point difference.

In **questionnaire 4** (June, 2006) an emphasis is put on 9 scores that occupy the scale between 1.00–2.00, only one trait – distressed, appears between 2.00–3.00 with the value of 2.50, comparing questionnaire 1; it circulates around 3.85 with the difference of 1.35. The lowest means are represented by guilty: 1.25 and upset, hostile, irritable, afraid that appear with the same score – 1.38. It indicates that all trait scores are involved in the decreasing zone within the lowest rate above 1.00.

Table 11. Mean scores of negative affects – group 2

Negative Affects – group 2										
	distressed	**upset**	**guilty**	**scared**	**hostile**	**irritable**	**ashamed**	**nervous**	**jittery**	**afraid**
questionnaire 1	4.00	4.00	1.75	4.13	1.75	3.88	3.13	3.88	3.63	3.88
questionnaire 2	3.38	2.50	1.63	3.00	1.63	2.88	2.38	2.63	2.63	3.00
questionnaire 3	3.00	1.88	1.50	2.13	1.63	1.88	2.00	1.88	1.50	2.38
questionnaire 4	2.50	1.38	1.25	1.88	1.38	1.38	1.50	1.63	1.50	1.38

In figure 45, all trait scores indicate a decreasing tendency within the mean scores, with the highest differences for upset: 4.00:1.40, scared: 4.10:1.90, irritable: 3.80:1.40, nervous: 3.80:1.60, jittery: 3.60:1.50 and afraid: 3.80:1.40. The lowest level of decrease is seen for guilty: 1.70:1.25 and hostile: 1.70:1.40. The indicators of distressed and ashamed cover the mid position with means of 4.00:2.50 and 3.10:1.50.

Figure 45. Negative affect changes – group 2

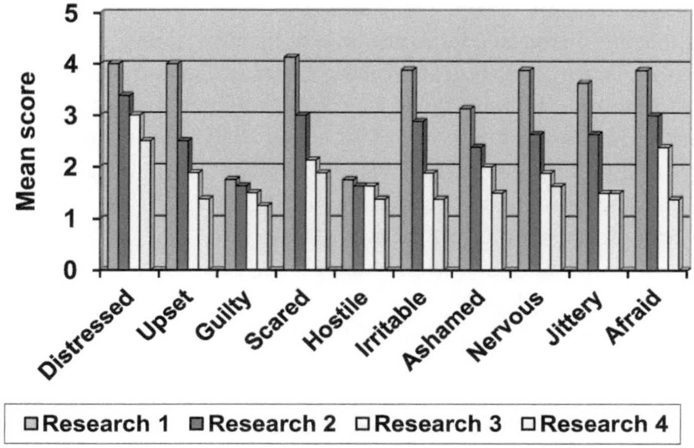

Groups 1 and 2 indicate a decreasing tendency of all negative affects.

Herman's indicator of negative affects (Oleś, 1992) shows 53% decrease – 18.2. The highest score difference circulates around 8.40 between research 1 and 2. The midlevel is achieved between 2 and 3 and equals 5.80; the lowest area is covered by 4.00, between 3 and 4. Almost the same – 50% decrease is clearly visible in group 1 (Table 12).

Table 12. The level of the intensity of negative affects – group 2

Intensity of negative affects			
R 1	R 2	R 3	R 4
34.0	25.6	19.8	15.8

R1 – Research 1

GROUP 3 (control)

Questionnaire 1 (September, 2005) presents the highest scores for nervous: 4.13, jittery: 4.00 and distressed: 3.75. The average values are covered by scared: 3.50, upset: 3.25 and afraid: 3.00. The lowest area is indicated by hostile: 1.75 and guilty: 2.00. The mode is high and circulates around 3.5. 2 scores are between 5.00–4.00, 4 means are located within 4.00–3.00, 3 values occupy the zone between 3.00–2.00 and 1 item fluctuates around 2.00–1.00.

Questionnaire 2 (December, 2005) depicts the intensity of negative affects that circulate around the highest scores of jittery: 4.13, nervous: 3.88 and scared, distressed: 3.63. The lowest scores appear in connection with hostile: 2.13, guilty: 2.63, irritable: 2.75 and afraid: 2.88. Comparing two questionnaires, it is worth noticing that any decreasing tendency does not appear. Jittery, ashamed, hostile, scared, guilty, upset present the increasing values, compared with research 1.

Questionnaire 3 (March, 2006) confirms accidental changes, with the highest means of jittery: 4.13, nervous: 3.75, upset: 3.50. 6 scores exist within the intensity level of 4.00–3.00, and 3 values correlate with 3.00–2.00. The mode covers 3.50 (the same item in questionnaire 1). The increase in the intensity is seen through irritable: 2.75:3.38 and guilty: 2.63:3.00. The means that sustain the level of intensity in questionnaires 2 and 3 are upset: 3.50:3.50, hostile: 2.13:2.13 and jittery: 4.13:4.13.

In **questionnaire 4** (June, 2006), 5 scores indicate an increasing tendency for the intensity of negative affects – distressed: 3.38:3.63, hostile: 2.13:2.25, irritable: 3.38:3.63, nervous: 3.75:4.50 and afraid: 2.75:3.63. The highest values are seen through nervous: 4.50, jittery: 4.00, irritable and afraid: 3.63. The lowest scores cover hostile and ashamed: 2.25. 1 value trait – ashamed is observed on the same level of the intensity in questionnaires 3 and 4 – 2.25. 4 means are in decrease: upset, guilty, scared and jittery.

Table 13. Mean scores of negative affects – group 3

Negative Affects – group 3										
	distressed	**upset**	**guilty**	**scared**	**hostile**	**irritable**	**ashamed**	**nervous**	**jittery**	**afraid**
questionnaire 1	3.75	3.25	2.00	3.50	1.75	2.88	2.88	4.13	4.00	3.00
questionnaire 2	3.63	3.50	2.63	3.63	2.13	2.75	3.25	3.88	4.13	2.88
questionnaire 3	3.38	3.50	3.00	3.00	2.13	3.38	2.25	3.75	4.13	2.75
questionnaire 4	3.63	3.13	2.63	2.75	2.25	3.63	2.25	4.50	4.00	3.63

Figure 46 demonstrates a decreasing tendency for two affects – scared and ashamed; the rest do not indicate any decreasing option. It is worth emphasising that all cases fluctuate permanently but such fluctuations are accidental, and cannot be logically explained.

Figure 46. Negative affect changes – group 3

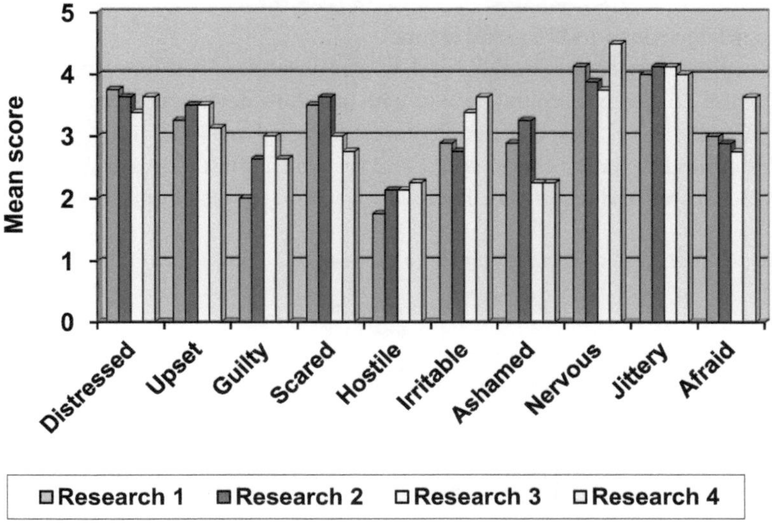

The level of negative affects (Oleś, 1992) starts with a 31.1 rate and finishes with 32.4; it indicates almost the same intensity with about 1-point increasing tendency. The differences between research 1 and 4 are almost not visible and oscillate on the same level of intensity (Table 14).

Table 14. The level of the intensity of negative affects – group 3

Intensity of negative affects			
R 1	R 2	R 3	R 4
31.1	32.4	31.3	32.4

R1 – Research 1

Comparing questionnaires 1 and 4, it ought to be noticed that the mean scores do not indicate the decreasing tendency of the intensity of negative affects. The changes are accidental. The initial and final values of 5 affects confirm the increase in the intensity of negative activation. 1 score – jittery – is seen on the same level of 4.00. 4 means appear with very little decrease: distressed, upset, scared, and ashamed, ranging from 0.12 to 0.63.

The Box and Whiskers plots for negative affects show a distinct presentation of trait scores of 4 questionnaires in 3 groups, seen through calculations of means, standard deviations and standard errors.

Box plot 47 analyses research 1 and divides negative affects into 2 groups: first, guilty and hostile as a separate group with standard deviations between 1.0 and 2.7, then distressed, upset, scared, irritable, ashamed, nervous, jittery and afraid, with standard deviations between 2.1 and 4.6. The highest scores are achieved by nervous, scared and distressed. The lowest ones are covered by guilty and hostile.

Figure 47. The Box and Whiskers plot for negative affects – research 1

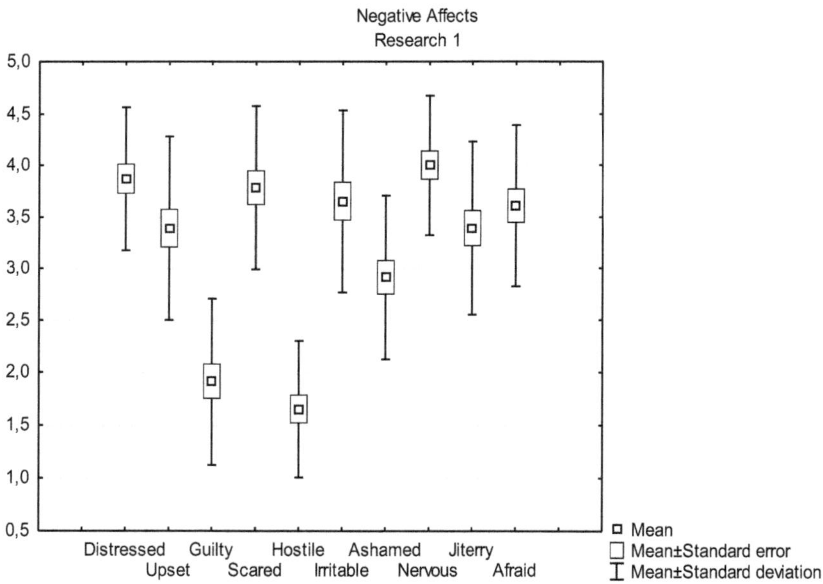

Research 2 presented in box plot 48 indicates a decreasing tendency for negative affects, with standard deviations starting from 0.8 to 4.2. The lowest scores are still covered by guilty and hostile; they create a group of affects but not so distinctly separated from other items. The highest values – distressed, irritable and jittery – are seen on a lower level than the ones achieved in research 1. The difference between R1 and R2 is on 0.3 level in connection with the lowest values, and 0.4 with the highest scores.

Figure 48. The Box and Whiskers plot for negative affects – research 2

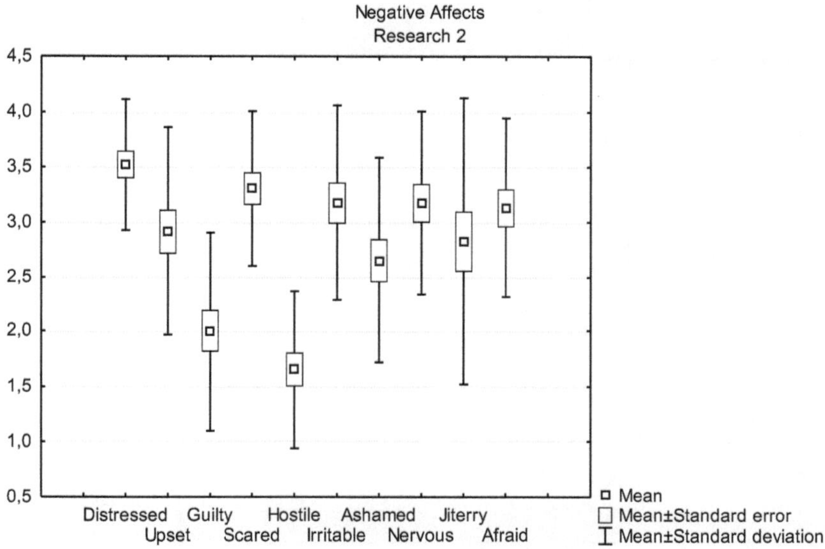

The box plot related to research 3 correlates with the values that fluctuate around 0.9–4.0 within one level of the intensity. The lowest standard deviations are represented by hostile and jittery, at about 0.9. The mid position values are equal the highest scores and are seen through upset, guilty, scared, irritable, nervous and jittery. The difference between R1 and R2 corresponds with the highest value of one affect – nervous: 4.0, equalling 0.2. Most affects occupy the 3.9–1.75 area. It is essential to emphasise that the standard deviations are permanently decreasing.

Figure 49. The Box and Whiskers plot for negative affects – research 3

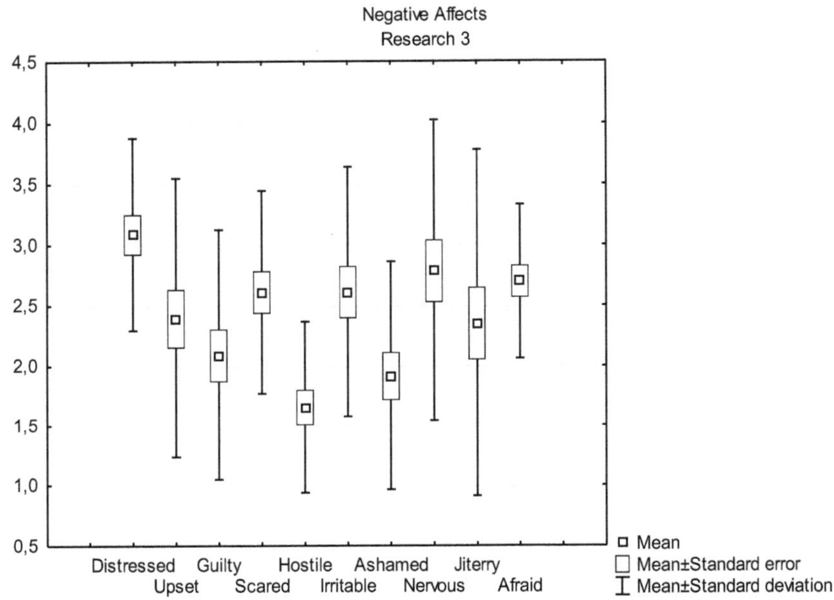

Research 4 analysed in box plot 50 correlates with the values around 2.0, in comparison with R1, it circulates around 3.5, with 1.5-point difference. The lowest scores – upset, guilty, hostile, nervous and jittery – are found on the 0.7 level, whereas the highest value, nervous, covers 0.9–4.0 (R1=4.7–3.4). A decreasing tendency of negative affects is clearly seen on the box plot.

Figure 50. The Box and Whiskers plot for negative affects – research 4

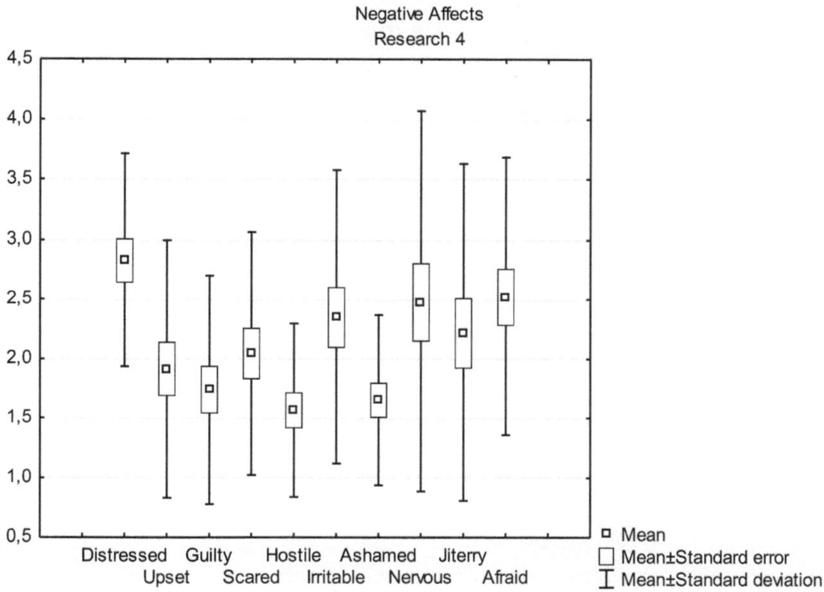

<u>Research hypothesis 3: The PLT influences language communicative competences.</u>

Independent variable: visual impairment
Dependent variable: achievements in L2

Each group covered 3 tests in L2:
1. Group 1: (1) September 2004, (2) January 2005, (3) June 2005.
2. Group 2: (1) September 2005, (2) January 2006, (3) June 2006.
3. Group 3: (1) September 2005, (2) January 2006, (3) June 2006.

Group 1

Tests 1–3 indicate language progress, related to building communicative competences in English during the PLT. Test 1 – a placement test – analyses values that fluctuate from 0–9 points; test 2: 20–28 points and test 3: 24–30 points evaluate the achievements in L2 during the PLT. Test 1 correlates with the mean of 5.14 and standard deviation equal 3.76. In test 2 the mean is 23.43 and standard deviation 2.82, and finally test 3 has a mean score of 27.43 and a standard deviation of 2.44. The highest rate is reached in test 2 and equals 18.29; the lowest mean difference appears in test 3 and focuses on 4.0. The total value of achievements in L2 equals 22.29. The values confirm hypothesis 3 – the PLT influences the achievements in L2.

Group 2
Test 1 scores oscillate between 0–10 points, test 2: 20–26 points and test 3: 23–30 points. The initial mean score equals 3.75 with SD=3.81. The final score (test 3) circulates within the mean of 26.25 and SD=2.38. The highest mean difference is visible in test 2 at 19.25. The lowest rate of language progress appears in test 3 at 3.25, the total mean difference is 22.50. The rate of achievement in L2 in test 2 covers almost the same value of 22.29 (comparing group 1). The value difference between the two groups circulates around 0.21, indicating linguistic progress within the PLT.

Group 3 (control)
The scores of test 1 define the boundaries between 0–9 points, test 2: 18–23, test 3: 20–25 points. The initial mean value is 5.88, SD=2.95 and the final one is related to 22.75 with SD=1.67. The highest indicator of achievement is seen in test 2 and equals 14.50. The lowest value is seen in test 3 and covers 2.37. The total score difference correlates with 16.87. Groups 1 and 2 represent higher scores than group 3. The rate of achievement in group 3 is lower than in groups 1 and 2 but still confirms the language progress.

Table 15. The scores achieved in L2 in three groups

	Research	Mean	Standard Deviation	Minimum	Maximum
Group 1	R 1	5,14	3,76	0,0	9,0
	R 2	23,43	2,82	20,0	28,0
	R 3	27,43	2,44	24,0	30,0
Group 2	R 1	3,75	3,81	0,0	10,0
	R 2	23,00	2,14	20,0	26,0
	R 3	26,25	2,38	23,0	30,0
Group 3	R 1	5,88	2,95	0,0	9,0
	R 2	20,38	1,69	18,0	23,0
	R 3	22,75	1,67	20,0	25,0

The scores achieved in tests 1–3 do not cover a normal distribution, so for differentiation between the values of the tests, it was essential to use a Kruskal-Wallis test (Greń, 1984). The mean in test 1 is exactly the same in the three groups. Crucial differences appear in connection with the comparison of data in tests 2 and 3. The scores of test 2 do not indicate significant differences between groups 1–3. For test 3 the noticeable difference covers the scores between groups 3 and 1 (p=0,005) and between groups 3 and 2 (p=0.033). It confirms that the values observed in group 3 are relatively lower than in groups 1 and 2.

Table 16. Kruskal-Wallis test for difference recognition

Dependent variable	H	p
Test 1	1,246	0,536
Test 2	6,630	0,036
Test 3	11,484	0,003

Figure 51 presents test achievements in L2. Groups 1 and 2 develop in parallel with a clear distinction associated with group 3. The highest progress appears between test 1 and 2, the lowest is seen between tests 2 and 3. The highest indicator of language development is covered by group 1. The starting points indicating the level of English before the PLT have their sources around 5.0, and after the psycho-linguistic therapy, they are rooted around the mean score equalling 27.

Figure 51. L2 test evaluation

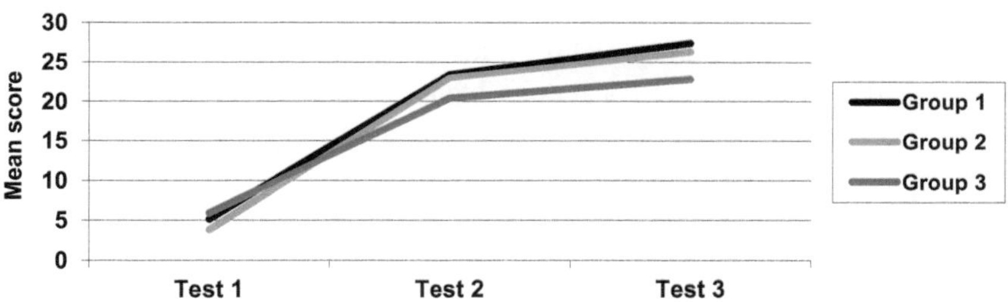

Box plot 52 presents three groups; the initial scores between 5.0–7.0 are the highest in relation to group 3. The lowest values are associated with group 2 and occupy the area between 2.5–5.0. Group 1 correlates with the average scores between 4.0–6.0. Group 1 and 2 create the same field of language competences. Group 3 is found as "withdrawn", in comparison with groups 1 and 2.

Figure 52. The Box and Whiskers plot for achievements in L2 – test 1

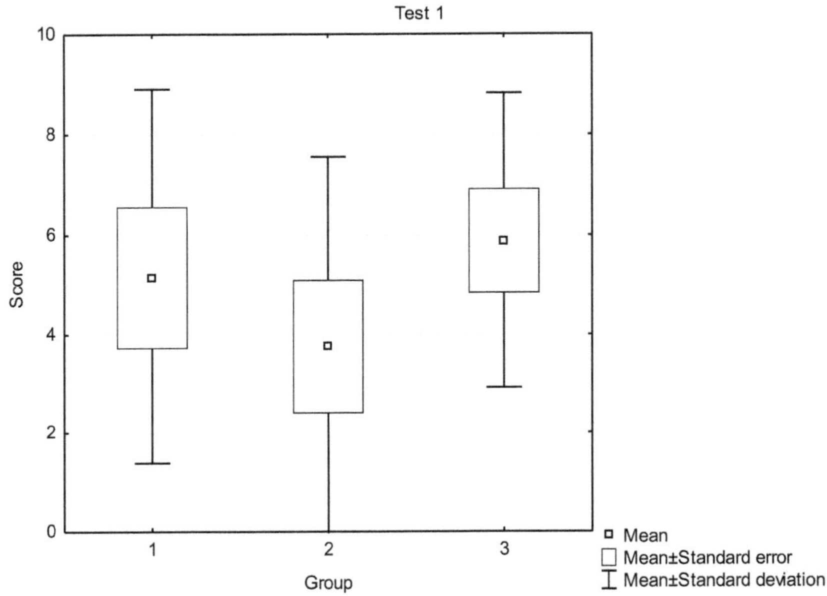

Box plot 53 presents test 2 scores, within two levels of achievements in L2, one encompassing groups 1 and 2 and the other related to group 3. The test clearly indicates that groups 1 and 2 achieve a higher level in L2; group 3 is seen as noticeably separated from 1 and 2. The rates in groups 1 and 2 circulate around 22.0–24.5; the indicators for group 3 are found between 21.0–20.0 which suggests a lower level of achievement in L2 with a 3.5 rate difference.

Figure 53. The Box and Whiskers plot for achievements in L2 – test 2

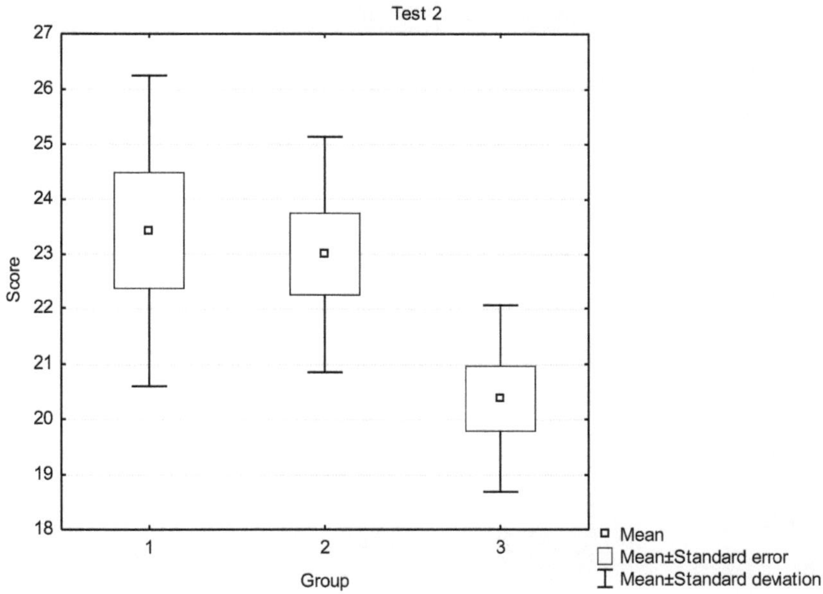

The achievements in L2 in test 3 (Figure 54) are seen through two-layered building. One layer is represented by groups 1 and 2 (the same in box plot 53) and the other is created by group 3. Groups 1 and 2 circulate around 25.0–28.0, and group 3 around 22.0–23.0. As it has been emphasised, the PLT influences language communicative competences more effectively in groups 1 and 2 than it is acquired in the control group, which indicates a lower rate of linguistic development.

Figure 54. The Box and Whiskers plot for achievements in L2 – test 3

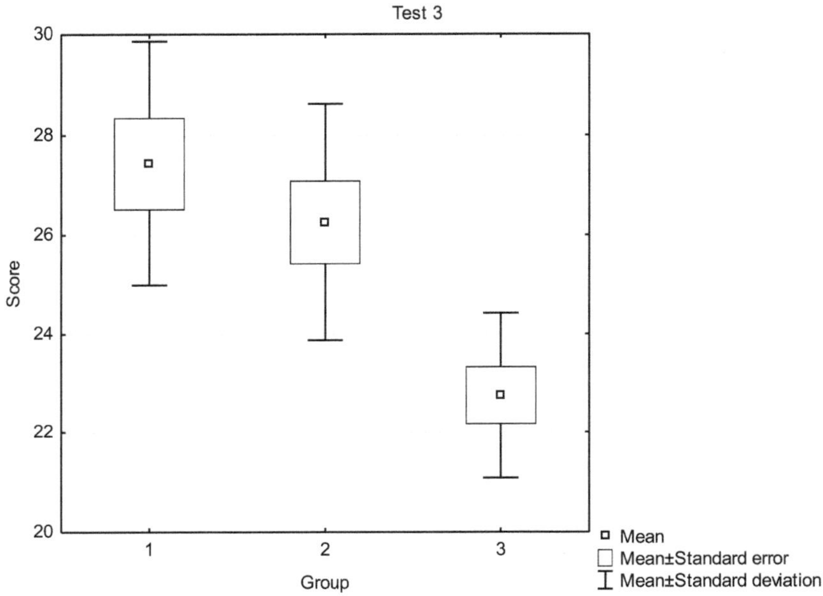

6.7. A Mann-Whitney U test

To verify the findings on the differences between groups 1 and 2, and 2 with 3, a Kolmogorov-Smirnov test was used to confirm the impression that scores were not normally distributed.

A two-sample Kolmogorov-Smirnov test is a nonparametric method for comparing two samples, as it is sensitive to differences in both location and shape of the empirical cumulative distribution functions of two groups. Kolmogorov lambda equals 0,178 and $p<0,01$, therefore a Mann-Whitney's U test was found useful (Greń, 1984). The U test evaluates if the medians between two groups differ significantly. To conduct the Mann-Whitney U test, each group must have scores on two variables, the grouping variable (independent) and the test variable (dependent). U value is compared to the table of critical values for U, based on the sample size of each group. If U exceeds the critical value at some significant level (usually equals 0.05), it means that it is evidence to reject a null hypothesis (H0) in favour of an alternative hypothesis (H1). Under a null hypothesis the distributions of both groups are equal, so that the probability of an observation from one population (X) exceeding an observation from the second population (Y) equals the probability of an observation from Y exceeding an observation from X, so that is there is a symmetry between groups 1 and 2. Under an alternative hypothesis, distributions of both groups are different.

I used the Mann-Whitney test and obtained p values less than 0.05. I evaluated the mean ranks of the intensity of affects for groups 1 and 2, and for groups 2 and 3.

6.7.1. The comparison between groups 1 and 2

The Mann-Whitney U test was conducted to evaluate a null hypothesis and alternative 1 within groups 1 and 2:

H0: Distributions of the intensity of positive and negative affects are equal in groups 1 and 2.
H1: Distributions of the intensity of positive and negative affects are different in groups 1 and 2.

Research 1 reveals crucial differences in evaluation of only two affects: upset, with $p=0.021$ and jittery, with $p=0.004$. The other emotions were seen by the students in the same way; if $p>0.05$ then **H0 cannot be rejected**. It is worth noticing that the mean scores in group 2 were higher in 13 traits. The following affects were higher in group 1: strong, guilty, enthusiastic, proud, irritable, alert and attentive with 4.0–18.0 mean difference. The U values within 11 items correlate around 20.0.

Table 17. The Mann-Whitney U test – research 1 (groups: 1 and 2)

	Group 1	Group 2	U	p
Interested	58,0	62,0	26,0	0,867
Distressed	53,0	67,0	25,0	0,779
Excited	53,5	66,5	25,5	0,779
Upset	36,0	84,0	8,0	0,021
Strong	65,0	55,0	19,0	0,336
Guilty	61,0	59,0	23,0	0,613
Scared	47,0	73,0	19,0	0,336
Hostile	49,0	71,0	21,0	0,463
Enthusiastic	62,0	58,0	22,0	0,536
Proud	65,0	55,0	19,0	0,336
Irritable	65,0	55,0	19,0	0,336
Alert	67,0	53,0	17,0	0,232
Ashamed	49,5	70,5	21,5	0,463
Inspired	45,5	74,5	17,5	0,232
Nervous	58,5	61,5	25,5	0,779
Determined	53,0	67,0	25,0	0,779
Attentive	69,0	51,0	15,0	0,152
Jittery	32,5	87,5	4,5	0,004
Active	56,0	64,0	28,0	1,000
Afraid	58,5	61,5	25,5	0,779

In research 2, differences are visible for only two affects: irritable with $p=0.021$ and jittery with $p=0.040$ (the same trait appeared in research 1), thus $p>0.05$ occupies 18 affects and **H0 is still accepted**. Group 2 indicates higher scores of upset, scared, irritable, nervous, attentive and afraid.

Table 18. The Mann-Whitney U test – research 2 (groups: 1 and 2)

	Group 1	Group 2	U	p
Interested	49,0	71,0	21,0	0,463
Distressed	59,0	61,0	25,0	0,779
Excited	41,5	78,5	13,5	0,094
Upset	60,5	59,5	23,5	0,613
Strong	59,5	60,5	24,5	0,694
Guilty	59,5	60,5	24,5	0,694
Scared	63,0	57,0	21,0	0,463
Hostile	45,5	74,5	17,5	0,232
Enthusiastic	43,5	76,5	15,5	0,152
Proud	43,5	76,5	15,5	0,152
Irritable	75,5	44,5	8,5	0,021
Alert	59,5	60,5	24,5	0,694
Ashamed	54,5	65,5	26,5	0,867
Inspired	42,0	78,0	14,0	0,121
Nervous	65,0	55,0	19,0	0,336
Determined	50,5	69,5	22,5	0,536
Attentive	71,5	48,5	12,5	0,072
Jittery	38,0	82,0	10,0	0,040
Active	40,0	80,0	12,0	0,072
Afraid	68,0	52,0	16,0	0,189

In research 3 all affect traits were evaluated in the same way, with $p>0.05$, and still **H0 is an accepted version;** it confirms that the PLT has almost the same influence on the intensity of positive and negative affects within groups 1 and 2.

The highest p-value corresponds with the affect 'interested' and equals 1,000 (Table 19).

Table 19. The Mann-Whitney U test – research 3 (groups: 1 and 2)

	Group 1	Group 2	U	p
Interested	56,0	64,0	28,0	1,000
Distressed	52,5	67,5	24,5	0,694
Excited	44,0	76,0	16,0	0,189
Upset	53,0	67,0	25,0	0,779
Strong	61,5	58,5	22,5	0,536
Guilty	62,0	58,0	22,0	0,536
Scared	70,0	50,0	14,0	0,121
Hostile	45,5	74,5	17,5	0,232
Enthusiastic	45,5	74,5	17,5	0,232
Proud	42,0	78,0	14,0	0,121
Irritable	71,5	48,5	12,5	0,072
Alert	65,5	54,5	18,5	0,281
Ashamed	47,5	72,5	19,5	0,336
Inspired	41,0	79,0	13,0	0,094
Nervous	70,5	49,5	13,5	0,094
Determined	40,0	80,0	12,0	0,072
Attentive	59,5	60,5	24,5	0,694
Jittery	50,0	70,0	22,0	0,536
Active	43,0	77,0	15,0	0,152
Afraid	68,5	51,5	15,5	0,152

Research 4 presents differences related to two affects: proud with p=0.021, and afraid with p=0.004. And again the same p-values appear above 0.05, suggesting that **H0 is still accepted**. 18 traits are seen in the similar or almost the same way confirming the PLT impact.

Table 20. The Mann-Whitney U test – research 4 (groups: 1 and 2)

	Group 1	Group 2	U	p
Interested	53,0	67,0	25,0	0,779
Distressed	50,0	70,0	22,0	0,536
Excited	52,5	67,5	24,5	0,694
Upset	49,5	70,5	21,5	0,463
Strong	62,0	58,0	22,0	0,536
Guilty	57,0	63,0	27,0	0,955
Scared	45,5	74,5	17,5	0,232
Hostile	45,5	74,5	17,5	0,232
Enthusiastic	50,0	70,0	22,0	0,536
Proud	36,0	84,0	8,0	0,021
Irritable	71,0	49,0	13,0	0,094
Alert	59,0	61,0	25,0	0,779
Ashamed	46,0	74,0	18,0	0,281
Inspired	46,0	74,0	18,0	0,281
Nervous	42,5	77,5	14,5	0,121
Determined	42,5	77,5	14,5	0,121
Attentive	46,5	73,5	18,5	0,281
Jittery	42,0	78,0	14,0	0,121
Active	51,0	69,0	23,0	0,613
Afraid	79,5	40,5	4,5	0,004

These are the following assumptions underlying the Mann-Whitney U test:

Assumption 1: The continuous distributions for the test variable are exactly the same for groups 1 and 2.

Assumption 2: The scores on the test variable are independent of each other. However, the distribution was continuous and has identical forms for two groups.

Overall, these data with $p>0.05$ observed in both groups suggest that they can be treated as parallel groups, with similar p-values and with the acceptance of the null hypothesis: H0 # H1; H0 cannot be rejected.

6.7.2. The comparison between groups 2 and 3

It was essential to compare groups 2 and 3 to provide confirmation of the hypotheses.

H0: Distributions of the intensity of positive and negative affects are equal in groups 2 and 3.

H1: Distributions of the intensity of positive and negative affects are different in groups 2 and 3.

Research 1 indicates two traits that are seen differently: irritable with p=0.015 and afraid with p=0.028. The rest of affects do not indicate any differences. The research results are similar in groups 1 and 2, with an emphasis on the initial version of the test. P-values indicate that the beginning point with H0 accepted is similar for three groups.

Table 21. The Mann-Whitney U test – research 1 (groups: 2 and 3)

	Group 2	Group 3	U	p
Interested	59,0	77,0	23,0	0,382
Distressed	74,0	62,0	26,0	0,574
Excited	54,5	81,5	18,5	0,161
Upset	84,0	52,0	16,0	0,105
Strong	70,0	66,0	30,0	0,878
Guilty	62,0	74,0	26,0	0,574
Scared	81,0	55,0	19,0	0,195
Hostile	68,0	68,0	32,0	1,000
Enthusiastic	72,0	64,0	28,0	0,721
Proud	59,0	77,0	23,0	0,382
Irritable	90,5	45,5	9,5	0,015
Alert	70,5	65,5	29,5	0,798
Ashamed	71,5	64,5	28,5	0,721
Inspired	68,0	68,0	32,0	1,000
Nervous	61,5	74,5	25,5	0,505
Determined	65,0	71,0	29,0	0,798
Attentive	69,0	67,0	31,0	0,959
Jittery	57,5	78,5	21,5	0,279
Active	66,0	70,0	30,0	0,878
Afraid	89,0	47,0	11,0	0,028

In research 2, seven differences appear for: enthusiastic – p=0.005, alert – p=0.000, nervous – p=0.007, determined – p=0.015, attentive – p=0.001, jittery – p=0.010, active – p=0.015. Research 2 indicates that differences are correlated with the experimental method used in the PLT; group 3 was not involved in the psycho-linguistic therapy. The scores indicate that H0 is not so distinctly accepted with an increasing tendency for trait differences with p<0.05.

Table 22. The Mann-Whitney U test – research 2 (groups: 2 and 3)

	Group 2	Group 3	U	p
Interested	85,0	51,0	15,0	0,083
Distressed	60,0	76,0	24,0	0,442
Excited	85,0	51,0	15,0	0,083
Upset	52,0	84,0	16,0	0,105
Strong	74,0	62,0	26,0	0,574
Guilty	50,5	85,5	14,5	0,065
Scared	53,5	82,5	17,5	0,130
Hostile	55,5	80,5	19,5	0,195
Enthusiastic	93,5	42,5	6,5	0,005
Proud	82,5	53,5	17,5	0,130
Irritable	70,5	65,5	29,5	0,798
Alert	99,5	36,5	0,5	0,000
Ashamed	52,5	83,5	16,5	0,105
Inspired	85,5	50,5	14,5	0,065
Nervous	43,5	92,5	7,5	0,007
Determined	91,0	45,0	9,0	0,015
Attentive	97,0	39,0	3,0	0,001
Jittery	44,0	92,0	8,0	0,010
Active	91,0	45,0	9,0	0,015
Afraid	71,0	65,0	29,0	0,798

Research 3 presents 13 affects seen differently in two groups: interested, excited, upset, guilty, enthusiastic, irritable, alert, inspired, nervous, determined, attentive, jittery, and active. Only 7 traits do not indicate differences. P-values tend to decrease below 0.05. At this stage, it confirms **H1 as a true hypothesis** for groups 2 and 3.

Table 23. The Mann-Whitney U test – research 3 (groups: 2 and 3)

	Group 2	Group 3	U	p
Interested	98,0	38,0	2,0	0,001
Distressed	60,5	75,5	24,5	0,442
Excited	98,0	38,0	2,0	0,001
Upset	42,5	93,5	6,5	0,005
Strong	72,5	63,5	27,5	0,645
Guilty	44,0	92,0	8,0	0,010
Scared	52,5	83,5	16,5	0,105
Hostile	55,5	80,5	19,5	0,195
Enthusiastic	97,0	39,0	3,0	0,001
Proud	84,5	51,5	15,5	0,083
Irritable	44,5	91,5	8,5	0,010
Alert	99,0	37,0	1,0	0,000
Ashamed	63,0	73,0	27,0	0,645
Inspired	98,0	38,0	2,0	0,001
Nervous	44,0	92,0	8,0	0,010
Determined	96,0	40,0	4,0	0,002
Attentive	97,0	39,0	3,0	0,001
Jittery	36,0	100,0	0,0	0,000
Active	100,0	36,0	0,0	0,000
Afraid	56,0	80,0	20,0	0,234

In research 4, only three affects: strong, scared and ashamed do not indicate differences. 17 emotions are seen differently with $p<0.05$ and **H1 is accepted**.

Table 24. The Mann-Whitney U test – research 4 (groups: 2 and 3)

	Group 2	Group 3	U	p
Interested	100,0	36,0	0,0	0,000
Distressed	46,0	90,0	10,0	0,021
Excited	97,0	39,0	3,0	0,001
Upset	39,0	97,0	3,0	0,001
Strong	80,5	55,5	19,5	0,195
Guilty	44,0	92,0	8,0	0,010
Scared	54,5	81,5	18,5	0,161
Hostile	47,5	88,5	11,5	0,028
Enthusiastic	100,0	36,0	0,0	0,000
Proud	98,0	38,0	2,0	0,001
Irritable	37,5	98,5	1,5	0,000
Alert	98,0	38,0	2,0	0,001
Ashamed	50,0	86,0	14,0	0,065
Inspired	100,0	36,0	0,0	0,000
Nervous	36,0	100,0	0,0	0,000
Determined	99,0	37,0	1,0	0,000
Attentive	100,0	36,0	0,0	0,000
Jittery	36,0	100,0	0,0	0,000
Active	98,0	38,0	2,0	0,001
Afraid	37,5	98,5	1,5	0,000

In essence, $p<0.05$, so H0 # H1; H1 is true. It can be assumed that the results indicate the difference in the intensity of positive and negative affects distributed in both groups; group 2 was loaded with the PLT issues and group 3 (control) worked with no PLT impact.

6.8. Discussion of the research results

The present study provides evidence for the fulfilment of three research hypotheses:

<u>Research hypothesis 1:</u> The PLT influences positive affects.
<u>Research hypothesis 2:</u> The PLT influences negative affects.
<u>Research hypothesis 3:</u> The PLT influences language communicative competences.

The findings collected in the case study confirm the influence of the psycholinguistic therapy "Touching the World" on the intensity of positive and negative affects of visually impaired students and the achievement in developing communicative competences in English.

Table 25 indicates that positive affects change from 1.3 to 4.4 (group 1), 1.2–4.5 (group 2) and negative affects change: group 1, 4.4–1.0; and group 2, 4.1–1.2. The initial modes of positive affects reach the boundaries of 1.00–2.00, with final ones equalling 3.00–5.00. The negative modes fluctuate around 3.00–5.00 in research 1 and indicate a decreasing tendency: 1.00–3.00 in research 4. Group 3 (control) does not show permanent positive or negative affect change measured during researches 1–4. The rates are almost on the same level of intensity or even tend to increase in negative activation.

Table 25. The mean scores for negative and positive affects

	Group 1				**Group 2**				**Group 3**			
	R1	**R2**	**R3**	**R4**	**R1**	**R2**	**R3**	**R4**	**R1**	**R2**	**R3**	**R4**
Interested	1,71	2,57	3,57	4,14	1,63	2,88	3,63	4,25	2,00	2,25	2,13	2,13
Distressed	3,85	3,57	2,86	2,29	4,00	3,38	3,00	2,50	3,75	3,63	3,38	3,63
Excited	1,29	2,14	3,00	3,57	1,38	2,88	3,50	3,75	1,88	2,00	2,00	2,13
Upset	2,86	2,71	1,71	1,14	4,00	2,50	1,88	1,38	3,25	3,50	3,50	3,13
Strong	2,00	2,43	2,71	3,14	1,63	2,25	2,38	2,88	1,50	2,00	2,13	2,25
Guilty	2,00	1,71	1,71	1,29	1,75	1,63	1,50	1,25	2,00	2,63	3,00	2,63
Scared	3,71	3,29	2,71	1,43	4,13	3,00	2,13	1,88	3,50	3,63	3,00	2,75
Hostile	1,43	1,14	1,14	1,00	1,75	1,63	1,63	1,38	1,75	2,13	2,13	2,25
Enthusiastic	1,71	2,57	3,43	4,29	1,50	3,13	3,88	4,50	1,38	2,00	2,25	2,38
Proud	1,57	1,86	2,29	2,57	1,25	2,38	2,88	3,63	1,63	1,75	2,00	1,75
Irritable	4,29	4,00	2,57	2,00	3,88	2,88	1,88	1,38	2,88	2,75	3,38	3,63
Alert	4,43	4,29	4,29	4,14	3,88	4,13	3,88	4,00	3,75	1,75	1,88	1,88
Ashamed	2,71	2,29	1,43	1,14	3,13	2,38	2,00	1,50	2,88	3,25	2,25	2,25
Inspired	1,28	2,43	3,29	4,14	1,75	3,00	4,00	4,50	1,75	2,38	2,00	1,88
Nervous	4,00	3,00	2,71	1,14	3,88	2,63	1,88	1,63	4,13	3,88	3,75	4,50
Determined	1,86	2,57	2,86	3,43	2,00	2,88	3,63	4,13	2,13	1,63	2,00	2,00
Attentive	4,43	4,29	3,86	3,71	3,75	3,63	3,75	4,13	3,63	2,00	2,25	1,63
Jittery	2,43	1,57	1,29	1,00	3,63	2,63	1,50	1,50	4,00	4,13	4,13	4,00
Active	1,43	2,00	2,71	3,57	1,50	2,88	3,25	3,75	1,50	1,63	1,75	1,63
Afraid	4,00	3,57	3,00	2,57	3,88	3,00	2,38	1,38	3,00	2,88	2,75	3,63

The research findings confirm the mean differences between research 1 and 4 in the positive and negative affects change (Table 26). Positive values indicate an increase in positive activation, whereas minus scores reflect a decrease in the intensity of negative affects. The highest increase in positive affects in group 1 is related to inspired: 2.86, enthusiastic: 2.57, interested: 2.43, excited: 2.29 and active: 2.14. The highest values in group 2 cover enthusiastic: 3.0, interested: 2.63, excited and proud: 2.38 and active: 2.25. Similar positive affects tend to rise in both groups. Group 3 presents lower rates of change; the highest rate of positive affects change is seen through enthusiastic (just one trait with the high rate): 1.0, excited and strong: 0.25 and interested: 0.13. The highest decrease in negative affect in group 1 correlates with nervous: -2.86, irritable: -2.29, upset: -1.71, distressed and ashamed: 1.57. The highest decrease in group 2 is visible through upset: -2.63, irritable, afraid: -2.50, scared, nervous: -2.25, jittery: -2.13. Group 3 represents the highest decrease in scared: -0.75, ashamed: -0.63. The values given above confirm that the increase in positive affects is noticeably found in groups 1–2 in all traits, and in group 3 just few trait scores indicate the change in affects. The lowest increase in positive affects in group 1 is related to strong: 1.14 and proud: 1.00, in group 2, attentive: 0.38 and alert: 0.13, and in group 3, interested, proud, inspired and active: 0.13. The lowest decrease in negative affects is found in group 1, hostile: -0.43, group 2, hostile: -0.38, and in group 3, distressed, upset: -0.12.

Table 26. The mean differences between research 1 and 4

	Group 1	Group 2	Group 3
Interested	2,43	2,63	0,13
Distressed	-1,57	-1,50	-0,12
Excited	2,29	2,38	0,25
Upset	-1,71	-2,63	-0,12
Strong	1,14	1,25	0,75
Guilty	-0,71	-0,50	0,63
Scared	-2,29	-2,25	-0,75
Hostile	-0,43	-0,38	0,50
Enthusiastic	2,57	3,00	1,00
Proud	1,00	2,38	0,13
Irritable	-2,29	-2,50	0,75
Alert	-0,29	0,13	-1,88
Ashamed	-1,57	-1,63	-0,63
Inspired	2,86	2,75	0,13
Nervous	-2,86	-2,25	0,38
Determined	1,57	2,13	-0,13
Attentive	-0,71	0,38	-2,00
Jittery	-1,43	-2,13	0,00
Active	2,14	2,25	0,13
Afraid	-1,43	-2,50	0,63

In essence, huge differences appear in groups 1 and 2. In group 3 changes are barely visible.

The change of affects is also clearly seen in Herman's pattern (Oleś, 1992) for measuring the intensity of positive and negative activation. The values indicate the increase in positive affects in groups 1 and 2, starting from 17.3 and 16.4, with the final scores of 32.6 and 35.5; it confirms hypothesis 1 related to the positive affect increase during the psycho-linguistic therapy "Touching the World". The scores associated with negative affects circulate around 30–31,3 (group 1) and 34.0 (group 2), verifying hypothesis 2 as true. The results of the control group and group 1 emphasise the affect change in connection with positive activation that oscillates almost on the same level at the initial stage of 17.4; the final values are 17.8 for the control group and 32.6 for group 1. The negative affect correlates with 31.1 at the beginning (research 1) and 32.4 in research 4, which indicates 1.3 increase in negative activation in the control group (Table 27).

The initial and final results of groups 1 and 2 indicate about 50% increase in positive affects and 50% decrease in negative ones; the values in the control group are still on the same level; the increase rate of positive activation is 0.04 that equals about 2% and 1.3 in negative affects – 4% (Table 27).

Table 27. The intensity of positive and negative affects

	Group 1				Group 2				Group 3			
	R1	R2	R3	R4	R1	R2	R3	R4	R1	R2	R3	R4
Positive	17,3	22,9	27,7	32,6	16,4	25,9	30,9	35,5	17,4	17,3	18,5	17,8
Negative	31,3	26,9	21,1	15,0	34,0	25,6	19,8	15,8	31,1	32,4	31,3	32,4

Comparing the results, I found it useful to evaluate the relation between positive and negative affects, using P/N indicator that demonstrates a dominant affect: positive or negative; if P/N<1 negative affects are dominant, if P/N >1, positive affects prevail. Groups 1 and 2 represent P/N >1, reached, but not in the same period of time. In group 1 – P/N=1.32 in research 3, after 6-month PLT and then P/N=1.67 after 10 months in research 4. In group 2 P/N=1.02 is achieved earlier after 3 months in research 2 and after 6 months, it occupies P/N=1.57 (research 3); finally, it correlates with P/N=2.11 indicating positive affects that prevail over negative ones; for each negative point, two points of positive affects are shown. It confirms that hypotheses 1 and 2 are true. Group 3 does not indicate PN>1, but P/N=0.65 in its initial value and final P/N=0.55 that correlate with the relation of negative affects over positive ones.

Table 28. The relation between affects

	Group 1				Group 2				Group 3			
	R1	R2	R3	R4	R1	R2	R3	R4	R1	R2	R3	R4
PR	0,36	0,46	0,57	0,68	0,33	0,50	0,61	0,69	0,36	0,35	0,37	0,35
NR	0,64	0,54	0,43	0,32	0,67	0,50	0,39	0,31	0,64	0,65	0,63	0,65
P/N	0,55	0,85	1,32	1,67	0,48	1,02	1,57	2,11	0,65	0,55	0,60	0,55

PR – an indicator of the intensity of positive affects
NR – an indicator of the intensity of negative affects
P/N – the relation between positive and negative affects
R1 – research 1

The dynamic path of positive affects is clearly demonstrated in figure 55. The beginning point indicates almost the same level of the intensity shared by three groups. Groups 1 and 2 show an increasing tendency for positive activation. In the control group, the level of the intensity does not indicate any change, it stays stable, on the same level, with no positive affects change.

Figure 55. The positive affect ratio

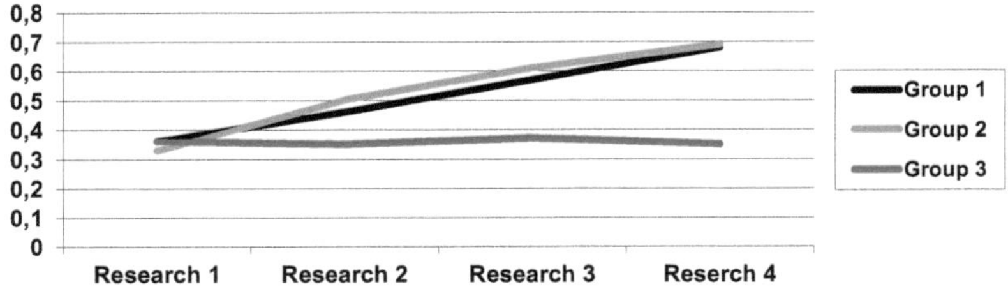

The fluctuations of negative affects indicate a noticeable decrease in the relation between groups 1 and 2; they are coherent in the intensity of their activation, with the highest values concerned with group 2. In group 3, the negative affect change is demonstrated through the initial and final scores concentrated on the same level of change. It should be noted that the beginning point is again shared by 3 groups, but within a two-path development (Figure 56).

Figure 56. The negative affect ratio

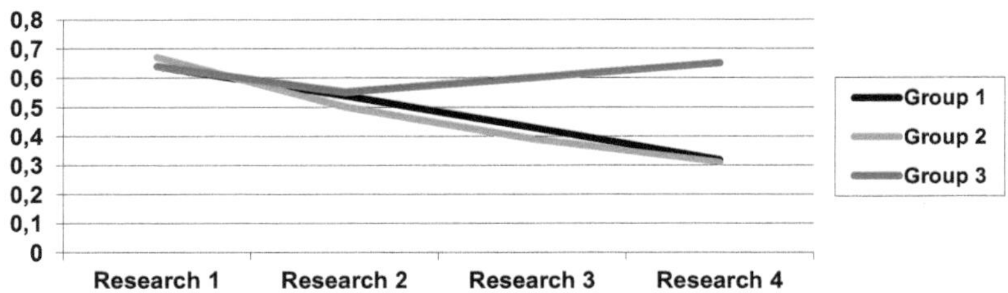

The achievements in L2 indicate the increase in communicative competences seen within two-layered recognition, first, within groups 1 and 2, and second, in group 3. The indicator of linguistic development is higher in groups 1 and 2. Group 3 shows the lower rate of language development. It should be noted that the initial point for the control group was the highest, whereas the final score was the lowest.

These results can be generalised due to the appropriate number of subjects involved in the psycho-linguistic therapy "Touching the World".

In conclusion, the research results revealed that hypotheses 1, 2 and 3 were true.

Chapter Seven: Conclusions and implications for further research

7.0. Introductory remarks

On the basis of the qualitative and quantitative results of the study, and the theoretical perspectives presented in the previous chapters, this chapter proposes recommendations for language teachers of visually impaired students. Furthermore, the implications for future research are outlined through current research findings.

7.1. Conclusions

Visually impaired students stimulated me to investigate the construction of a therapy based on three-layered involvement: disability–person–language. Psychological and physical consequences of the disorder – the issue of sensory compensation – were considered as crucial elements of the efficient and well-organised psycho-linguistic therapy "Touching the World". The therapy confirms the involvement of the humanistic approach to language teaching on the basis of the psychological development of the students. The PLT promotes self-growth and self-actualisation – the goal content – as the added value of the therapy. Overcoming barriers and helping people to release feelings lead students to increase their positive qualities of "self" such as joy, peace, and self-esteem. The PLT builds freedom on the basis of a mental overcoming of physical limitations of visual impairment through kinaesthetically involved techniques; the tactile experience of touching and manipulating sand and water provides the activation of self-expression. The implementation of diverse techniques impacts the students' central nervous systems, balancing the two hemispheres.

The results of the research indicate that the psycho-linguistic therapy "Touching the World" for visually impaired students is an effective model for increasing positive activation and decreasing negative affects. It also influences the students' linguistic competences. According to the therapy, language is seen as a therapeutic tool that "operates" not only on the linguistic layer but, predominantly, on the mental one of human being. On the one hand, the linguistic area is rooted in mental-layered recognition, and on the other, the mental field provides a fertile starting point for the PLT theory and practice. In all, both layers of language act in an efficient reciprocation.

The students, struggling with everyday life and with their disabilities, relished the journey of becoming more conscious about themselves, their inner world, and their relationships with others within the therapy. I hope that experience of flow was also shared by them.

In essence, the psycho-linguistic therapy "Touching the World" is an approach to the identity of the human being; an identity that is constructed, justified and maintained through language (Kroger, 2007).

7.2. Recommendations for language teachers of visually impaired students

The information and knowledge gained from the current research results allow me to generate specific suggestions for language as a therapeutic tool.

According to Tomkins (1962), optimal mental health requires maximisation of positive affects and minimisation of negative affects. It is essential that teachers of visually impaired students keep in mind that teaching a language can be regarded as a therapeutic tool that intensifies positive and decreases negative activation. Language cannot be considered separately without emotions that are tightly connected with a didactic process. Every teacher should be aware that teaching a foreign language to the visually impaired can influence their self-esteem development. Thus foreign language teachers should bear in mind that learners should become involved in the process of teaching-learning English, with accompanied feelings of mental and physical safety and independence, and with a set of clear goals to be achieved related to their abilities, aptitudes, and visual impairment.

The main goal should be enabling FL teachers to create a more supportive and appropriate classroom environment that will help students evoke linguistic competences. Students ought to be provided with a variety of techniques to intensify mental and linguistic input in parallel involvement through creative and hapticly effective tools. Furthermore, a facilitative environment in a foreign language classroom is an important factor in helping students to increase positive affects and decrease negative ones. Therefore, a foreign language classroom should be unobstructed by fear and anxiety. Most importantly, the relationships between the teacher and students, and within the group, play a fundamental function.

The next recommendation is that for the purpose of achieving the aforementioned goals teachers should be enthusiastic experts, understanding the degrees of blindness with passion and involvement, and thereby inducing positive affect experience within the subject they teach, which can serve as a model for their students to follow. Therefore, it can be concluded that the role of teachers' individual characteristics seems to be vital. Another crucial implication is that teachers should be able to maintain harmony between students' abilities and the challenges they are faced with. The students' goals must be clear and approachable. According to Williams and Burden (1997), when students are involved and concentrated, they are aware of their aims and they are worried neither about failure nor about challenging tasks. In an ideal situation a student should have the feeling of development by constant raising of skills. The steps of the teaching-learning process should be carefully graded.

It should be also noted that learners ought to have optimal control, providing them with opportunities to change the intensity of positive and negative affects.

To conclude, teachers' awareness of the degree of visual impairment, understanding students' background and the implementation of the appropriate multisensory training in the teaching-learning process will affect the usefulness of methods and techniques, influencing the affect change and linguistic development.

7.3. Implications for further research into pedagogy for the visually handicapped

These findings show how interaction in teaching practicum can be arranged so that students have opportunities to change their emotional level of positive and negative activation and develop linguistic competences.

The present study was devoted to language as an indicator of the intensity of positive and negative affects. In order to extend the findings, it is vital to focus on some implications for future research:

Implication 1
The implementation of one huge sandtray for a whole group.

Implication 2
Tactile structure repetition can be enriched with Braille.

Implication 3
"Vocabulary movement – the word segmentation technique" can be extended to one-syllable words to revise lexis.

Implication 4
The edu-kinaesthetic area by Dennison should be used to measure learning styles of visually impaired students.

Implication 5
Controlled breathing techniques helping relaxation should be a part of each English lesson.

Implication 6
The metronome listening can be used to learn polysyllabic words.

Implication 7
The PANAS questionnaire could be extended to "The Self-Confrontation Method" by Hermans.

Implication 8
The implementation of the sandtray therapy for the sighted, within the process of teaching-learning English.

Although these particular arrangements of the teaching-learning process to the visually impaired seem to have a powerful influence on the changes made in the intensity of affects and language acquisition, I am not presenting my findings as prescriptions for teachers of the visually handicapped. Rather, I would like to encourage English teachers to be aware of what powerful tools they hold in their hands. My suggestions to explore language as a therapy tool show how deeply the possibilities and discoveries are hidden in a language teaching-learning process. I emphasise this issue to empower English teachers to see teaching differently.

If English teachers believe that the purpose of teaching a foreign language is to understand the process going on in language acquisition of the visually handicapped, they cannot deny the relevance of this study.

References

Adler, G. (1924): *The practice and theory of individual psychology.* New York: Harcourt, Brace & Company.

Allan, J. (2007): *Jungian play therapy.* Paper presented at the Play Therapy Summer Institute, Center for Play Therapy, University of North Texas, Denton, Texas.

Allen, H. B. (ed.) (1965): *Teaching English as a second language.* New York: McGraw - Hill.

Allen, V. F. (1983): *Techniques in vocabulary teaching.* New York: Oxford University Press.

Allport, G. W. (1937): *Personality: A psychological interpretation.* New York: Holt.

Altman, J. (1970): *Biological bases of behaviour.* PWN.

Anastasi, A. (1982): *Psychological testing.* New York: Macmillan.

Arndt, W. B. (1974): *Theories of personality.* New York: Macmillan.

Austin, J. L. (1962): *How to do things with words.* Cambridge, Mass.: Harvard University Press.

Baddeley, A. (1983): *Your memory.* London: Penguin.

Badenoch, B. (2008): *Being a brain-wise therapist: A practical guide to interpersonal neurobiology.* New York: W. W. Norton & Company.

Bailliart, P. (1964): *Dziecko niewidome. Wychowanie, nauka, medycyna, socjologia.* Warszawa.

Bandler, R. – J. Grinder (1975): *The structure of magic.* Palo Alto: Science and Behaviour Books.

Bandler, R. (1985): *Using your brains for a change.* Moab, UT: Real People Press.

Bandura, A. (1990): "Self-efficacy: Toward a unifying theory of behavioural change", *Psychological Review* 84: 191–215.

Bardi, A. – S. H. Schwartz (2003): "Values and behavior: Strength and structure of relations", *Personality and Social Psychology Bulletin* 29: 1207–1220.

Barone, D. M. (2004): "Literacy research methodologies: Case study research", in: M. H., Mallette – N.K. Duke (eds.), 7–27, New York: Guilford Press.

Belin, P. – R. J. Zattorre – P. Lafaille – P. Ahad – B. Pike (2000): "Voice selective areas in human auditory cortex", *Nature* 403: 309–312.

Belzyt, J. (2012): *Niepełnosprawność - edukacja - dorosłość. Studium przypadku osoby ociemniałej.* Oficyna Wydawnicza "Impuls".

Berne, E. (1966): *Principles of group treatment.* New York: Oxford University Press.

Bertocci, P. A. (1988): *The person and primary emotions.* New York: Springer – Verlag.

Boeree, C. G. (2006): *Personality theories.* An Electronic Textbook. http://webspace.ship.edu/cgboeree/personcontents.html.

Bogdan, R. C. – S. K. Biklen (2006): *Qualitative research in education: An introduction to theory and methods.* Allyn & Bacon.

Bostock, P. (1972): *Dialogues and songs.* Walton-on-Thames: Nelson.

Bow, J. N. (1993): "Overcoming resistance: The therapeutic powers of play", in: Schaefer C. (ed.), 17–40, Northvale, NJ: Jason Aronson.

Brehm, J. W. (1999): "The intensity of emotions", *Personality and Social Psychology Review* 1, vol. 3: 2–22.

Brown, H. D. (1993): *Principles of language learning and teaching.* Englewood Cliffs, NJ: Prentice – Hall.

Brown, S. – C. Vaughan (2009): *Play: How it shapes the brain, opens the imagination, and invigorates the soul.* New York: Avery Books.

Brzeziński, J. (1978): *Metodologiczne i psychologiczne wyznaczniki procesu badawczego w psychologii.* UAM, Poznań.

Burklen, K. (1985): *Psychologia niewidomych.* Warszawa.

Buros, O. K. (1970): *Personality: tests and reviews.* The Gryphon Press, New Jersey.

Byrne, D. – S. Rixon (1982): *ELT Guide I: Communication Games.* London: NFER/Nelson/The British Council.

Cacioppo, J. T. – G. G. Berntson – J. T. Larsen – K. M. Poehlmann – T. A. Ito (2001): "Handbook of emotions: The psychophysiology of emotion", in Lewis M. – J. M. Haviland – Jones (eds.), 173–191, New York: The Guilford Press.

1995 *Callan Method. Teacher's handbook.* Orchard Publishing LTD.

Campbell, C. – H. Kryszewska (1995): *Learner-based teaching.* Oxford University Press.

Caplan, F. – T. Caplan (1974): *The power of play.* New York: Anchor Books.

Carroll, J. B. (1966): *Language and thought.* Eaglewood Cliffs. New York: Prentice – Hall.

Cassie, D. (1992): *So who's perfect! People with visible differences tell their own stories.* Scottdale, PA: Herald Press.

Cattell, R. B. (1946): *Description and measurement of personality.* New York: World Book.

Chomsky, N. (1968): *Language and mind.* New York: Harcourt Brace and World.

Christensen, L. B. (1997): *Experimental methodology.* Boston: Allyn & Bacon.

Chusid, J. G. (1996): *Structure and function in neurology.* Sage Thousand Oaks.

Creswell, J. W. (1998): *Qualitative Inquiry and Research Design. Choosing Among Five Traditions.* Sage Thousand Oaks, CA: Publications.

Csikszentmihalyi, M. (1993): *The evolving self: A psychology for the Third Millennium.* HarperCollins.

Csikszentmihalyi, M. (1996): *Creativity: flow and psychology of discovery and invention.* HarperCollins.

Csikszentmihalyi, M. (2008): *Flow: the psychology of optimal experience.* HarperCollins.

Czerwińska, K. (2006): "Możliwości wykorzystania grafiki dotykowej w nauczaniu języków obcych – teoria a praktyka", *Szkoła specjalna* 5: 323–329.

Czerwińska, K. (2007): "Zastosowanie wiedzy o umyśle w edukacji niewidomych", *Niepełnosprawność i Rehabilitacja* 2: 81–87.

Czerwińska, K. (2008): "Tyflografika w nauczaniu języków obcych – z doświadczeń projektu Per linguas mundi ad laborem", *Niepełnosprawność i Rehabilitacja* 2: 78–89.

Dakowska, M. (2005): *Teaching English as a foreign language. A guide for professionals.* Warszawa: Wydawnictwo Naukowe PWN.

Data, K. (2000): "W jaki sposób językoznawcy opisują emocje?", *Język a kultura* 2229, Wrocław.

Davis, P. – M. Rinvolucri (1987): *Relaxing dictations.* SEAL Newsletter.

Davitz, J. L. (1969): *The language of emotion.* New York: Academic Press.

De Bono, E. (1999): *Jak stosować myślenie lateralne. Rozwiązywanie problemów metodą pozalogiczną.* Warszawa: Medium.

Deci, E. L. – R. M. Ryan (2000): "Intrinsic and extrinsic motivations: Classic definitions and new directions", *Contemporary Educational Psychology* 25: 54–67.

De Domenico, G. (1995): *Sandtray world play: A comprehensive guide to the use of the sandtray in psychotherapeutic and transformational settings.* Oakland, CA: Vision Quest Images.

Deleuze, G. – F. Guattari (1987): *A thousand plateau.* Minneapolis: University of Minesota.

Demos, E. (ed.) (1995): *Exploring affect. The selected writings of Silvan S. Tompkins.* New York: Press Sindicate of the University of Cambridge.

Dennison, P. – G. Dennison (2003): *Gimnastyka mózgu.* Międzynarodowy Instytut Kinezjologii, Warszawa.

Denzin, N. K. (1984): *On understanding human emotion*. San Francisco: Jossey-Bass.

Dewey, J. (2007): *Moje pedagogiczne credo*. Warszawa.

Dorward, B. – N. Barraga (1968): *Teaching aids for blind and visually limited children*. American Foundation for The Blind, Inc. New York.

Douglas, T. (1983): *Groups: Understanding people together*. London: Tavistock Press.

Dubin, F. – E. Olshtain (1977): *Facilitating language learning: A Guidebook for the ESL/EFL Teacher*. New York: McGraw Hill.

Duffy, E. (1962): *Activation and behavior*. New York: Wiley.

Dulay, H. C. – M. K. Burt – S. Krashen (1982): *Language two*. New York: Oxford University Press.

Dunlop, F. (1977): "Human nature, learning and ideology", *The British Journal of Education Studies* XXV/3, October.

Dycht, M. (2005): *Koncepcja tyflopedagogiki w ujęciu Zofii Sękowskiej*, Wydawnictwo Salezjańskie, Warszawa.

Eichoff, L. (1952): "Dreams in sand", *Journal of Mental Science* 98: 235–243.

Ellis, A. (1962): *Reason and emotion in psychotherapy*. New York: Lyle Stuart.

Ellis, A. (2008): "Rational emotive behaviour therapy", in: Corsini R. – D. Wedding (eds.), *Current psychotherapies* 8: 187–222, Belmont, CA: Thomson.

Engler, B. (1985): *Personality theories*. Boston: Houghton Mifflin.

Erikson, E. H. (1978): *Adulthood*. New York: Norton.

Fonagy, P. – G. Gergely – E. Jurist – M. Target (2004): *Affect regulation, mentalization and the development of the self*. New York: Other Press.

Fraiberg, S. (1977): *Insights from the blind*. London: Souvenir Press.

Frank, Ch. – M. Rinvolucri (1983): *Grammar in action*. Oxford: Pergamon/ Munich: Max Hueber.

Fredrickson, B. L. (1998): "What good are positive emotions?", *Review of General Psychology* 2: 300– 319.

Freud, A. (1965): *The psycho-analytic treatment of children*. New York: International Universities Press.

Fridlund, A. J. (1992): "Darwin's anti-Darwinisms in the expression of the emotions in man and animals", *International Review of Studies on Emotion* 2: 117–138, Chichester: Wiley.

Frijda, N. H. (1986): *The emotions*. Cambridge: Cambridge University Press.

Gairns, R. – S. Redman (1986): *Working with words*. Cambridge University Press.

Gale, A. – A. J. Chapman (1984): *Psychology & social problems. An introduction to applied psychology*. John Wiley & Sons.

Gardner, H. (1993): *Multiple intelligences: the theory of practice*. New York: Basic Books.

Gardner, R. C. (1972): *Attitudes and motivation in second language learning*. Rowley, Mass: Newbury House Publishers, Inc.

Gatchel, R. J. – F. G. Mears (1982): *Personality theory, assessment and research*. St. Martin's Press – New York.

Gibbs, G. I. (1974): *Handbook of games and simulations*. London.

Gilligan, S. G. – G. H. Bower (1984): "Emotions, cognition and behavior: Cognitive consequences of emotional arousal", in: Izard, C. – J. Kagan – R. Zajonc (eds.), New York: Cambridge University Press.

Gougoux, F. – P. Belin – P. Voss – F. Lepore – M. Lassonde – R. J. Zattorre (2009): "Voice perception in blind persons: A functional magnetic resonance imaging study". *Neuropsychologia* 47: 2967–2974.

Grabias, S. (1981): *O ekspresywności języka*. Lublin.

Gregg, K. (1984): "Krashen's monitor and Occam's razor", *Applied Linguistics* 5: 79–100.

Greń, J. (1984): *Statystyka matematyczna. Modele i zadania*. Warszawa: PWN.

Gronlund, N. E. (2002): *Assessment of student achievement*. Boston: Allyn & Bacon 1998.

Gross, J. J. (ed.) (2009): *Handbook of emotion regulation*. The Guilford Press: New York – London.

Grundy, P. (2004): *Beginners*. Oxford University Press.

Gulliksen, H. (1950): *Theory of mental tests*. New York: Wiley.

Hadfield, J. (2002): *Classroom Dynamics*. Oxford University Press.

Hainninen, K. (1990): *Teaching the visually handicapped*. London.

Hannaford C. (1998): *Zmyślne ruchy, które doskonalą umysł*. Polskie Stowarzyszenie Kinezjologów, Warszawa.

Hancock, M. (2003): *English pronunciation in use*. Cambridge.

Hannan, J. (1989): "Easing students into dictogloss", *TEA News*: vol. 7, no. 1.

Hare, P. A. (1982): *Creativity in small groups*. London: Sage Publications.

Harmer, J. (1974): *English tea*. London: Macmillan.

Harmer, J. (2004): *The practice of English language teaching*. Longman.

Hatch, E. – C. Brown (1995): *Vocabulary, semantics, and language education*. Cambridge University Press.

Heszen – Niejódek, I. (1979): *Poznawcze uwarunkowania zachowania wobec własnej choroby.* Wrocław: Ossolineum.

Homeyer, L. E. – D. S. Sweeney (2011): *Sandtray therapy. A practical manual.* New York: Routledge Taylor & Francis Group.

Howatt, A. P. R. (1984): *A history of English language teaching.* Oxford: Oxford University Press.

Hug – Hellmuth, H. (1921): "On the technique of child-analysis", *International Journal of Psychoanalysis* 2: 287–305.

Izard, C. E. (1991): *The psychology of emotions.* New York: Plenum.

Jackson, S. L. (2009): *Research methods and statistics: A critical thinking approach. Jak świata mniej widzę: zaburzenia widzenia a jakość życia,* pod red. P. Olesia, S. Steuden i J. Toczołowskiego, Lublin: Towarzystwo Naukowe KUL, 2002.

Jung. C. G. (1977): *Symbols of transformation.* Princeton, NJ: Princeton University Press.

Kalff, D. (1980): *Sandplay, a psychotherapeutic approach to the psyche.* Santa Monica, CA: Sigo Press.

Kazdin, A. E. (1980): *Behaviour modification in applied settings.* Homewood, Ill.: Dorsey Press.

Kelly, G. (2004): *How to teach pronunciation.* Longman.

Klein, M. (1932): *The psycho-analysis of children.* London: Hogarth Press.

Kleinmuntz, B. (1967): *Personality measurement: An introduction.* Homewood, Ill.: Dorsey Press.

Kopka, S. (2002): *"Rzucać – co, czym, kto, kogo?".* Kraków: Universitas.

Krashen, S. – R. Scarcella (1978): "On routines and patterns in language acquisition and performance", *Language Learning* 28: 283–300.

Krashen, S. – T. Terrell (1983): *The natural approach: language acquisition in the classroom.* Hayward, CA: Alemany Press.

Krashen, S. (1985): *The input hypothesis.* London: Longman.

Krause, C. A. (1916): *The Direct Method in modern languages.* New York.

Kroger, J. (2007): *Identity development. Adolescence through adulthood.* London: Sage.

Krzeszowski, T. P. (1984): *Gramatyka angielska dla Polaków.* Warszawa.

Krzeszowski, T. P. (1993): *Gdy dziecko niedowidzi.* Bydgoszcz.

Krzeszowski, T. P. (1997): *Angels and devils in hell. Elements of axiology in semantics.* Warszawa: Wydawnictwo Energeia.

Krzeszowski, T. P. (2012): "Learning from the blind", in: *Foreign language didactics and its application in the educational setting.* SWSPiZ Łódź – Warszawa.

Kumaravadivelu, B. (2006): *Understanding language teaching.* Hillsdale: Lawrence Erlbaum.

Kurcz, I. (1976): *Psycholingwistyka*. Warszawa.

Leech, G. (1990): *Semantics. The study of meaning.* England: Penguin Books Ltd.

Leontiev, A. A. (1981): *Psychology and the language process.* Oxford: Pergamon Press.

Lewandowski, P. (2005): *Samoleczenie metodą BSM*. Warszawa.

Lewis, M. (1993): *The lexical approach*. LPT.

Lewis, M. – J. M. Haviland – Jones (ed.) (2001): *Handbook of emotions*. New York: The Guilford Press.

Littlewood, W. (1995): *Foreign and second language learning.* Cambridge University Press.

Llewelyn, S. (1989): "The dictogloss procedure and grammatical consciousness-raising: classroom-based research", *Prospect,* vol. 5, no. 1.

Lowenfeld, M. (1950): "The nature and use of the Lowenfeld World Technique in work with children and adults", *The Journal of Psychology* 30: 325–331.

Lozanov, G. (1978): *Suggestology and outlines of suggestopedy*. New York: Gordon and Breach Science Publishers.

Luria, A. R. (1975): *The mind of mnemonist*. London: Penguin.

Lyons, W. (1980): *Emotion*. Cambridge: Cambridge University Press.

Maddi, S. R. (1976): *Personality theories.* Homewood, Ill.: Dorsey.

Maia, B. H. M.S. (1998): "The language of emotion – metaphors, scenarios or metalanguage?", in Lewandowska – Tomaszczyk, B. (ed.), *Lexical semantics, cognition and philosophy,* Łódź University Press.

Maj, W. (1981): *Specifity of teaching foreign languages to blind Poles. Nauczanie niewidomych języków obcych z uwzględnieniem specyfiki polskiej*. Praca magisterska.

Majewski, T. (1983): *Psychologia niewidomych i niedowidzących.* Polskie Wydawnictwo Naukowe.

Marek, B. (2001): "Razem czy osobno? Integracyjne pomoce dydaktyczne w nauczaniu języków obcych", *Języki Obce w Szkole* 7: 93–102.

Marek, B. (2006): "Świat bez wzroku: wyzwania i rozwiązania w nauczaniu języka angielskiego osób niewidomych", w: J. Krieger-Knieja, U. Paprocka-Piotrowska (red.), *Komunikacja językowa w społeczeństwie informacyjnym. Nowe wyzwania dla dydaktyki języków obcych,* s. 64–75. Lublin: Towarzystwo Naukowe KUL.

Marieb, E. – K. Hoehn (2007): *Human anatomy and physiology.* Pearson Benjamin Cummings: San Francisco.

Maslow, A. H. (1943): "A preface to motivation theory", *Psychosomatic Medicine* 5: 85–92.

Maslow, A. H. (1970): *Motivation and personality.* New York: Harper and Row.

May, R. (1996): *Psychology and the human dilemma.* New York: Norton.

McAdams, D. P. (1996): "Personality, modernity and the storied self: A contemporary framework for studying persons", *Psychological Inquiry* 7: 295–321.

McDougall, W. (1928): "Feelings and emotions: Emotion and feeling distinguished", in: Reymert M. L. (ed.), Worcester: Clark University Press.

McLeish, J. (1973): *The Psychology of the learning group.* London: Hutchinson.

Merdinger, P. – J. Rosenfeld (1984): *Even if you can't carry a tune: grammar through popular songs.* Rowley, Mass.: Newbury House.

Mills, J. – R. Crowley (1986): *Therapeutic metaphors for children and the child within.* New York: Brunner/Mazel.

Mitchell, R. – F. Myles (2002): *Second language learning theories.* Cambridge University Press.

Morgan, J. – M. Rinvolucri (1997): *Vocabulary.* Oxford University Press.

Moskowitz, G. (1978): *Caring and sharing in the foreign language classroom.* Rowley, Mass.: Newburry House.

Murphey, T. (1996): *Music & song.* Oxford University Press.

Murphy, G. (1966): *Personality.* New York: Basic.

Murray, H. A. (1938): *Explorations in personality.* New York: Oxford University Press.

Myers, A. (1980): *Experimental psychology.* New York. Van Nostrand.

Norris, N. (1972): *Aims and methods in the teaching of English to the visually handicapped.* Birmingham RCEVH.

Nowakowska – Kempna I. (1995): *Konceptualizacja uczuć w języku polskim. Prolegomena.* Wyższa Szkoła Pedagogiczna Towarzystwa Wiedzy Powszechnej. Warszawa.

Nęcka, E. (2001): *Psychologia twórczości.* Gdańsk.

Oatley, K. (1992): *Best laid schemes.* Cambridge: Cambridge University Press.

Obuchowski, K. (1995): *Przez galaktykę potrzeb. Psychologia dążeń ludzkich.* Poznań: Zyski S-ka Wydawnictwo.

Oleś, P. (1992): *Metoda konfrontacji z sobą Huberta J. M. Hermansa.* Pracownia Testów Psychologicznych PTP. Warszawa.

Palmer, F. R. (1995): *Semantics.* Cambridge University Press.

Paluchowski, W. J. (2006): *Diagnoza psychologiczna. Podejście jakościowe i ilościowe*. Warszawa.

Papez, J. W. (1937): "A proposed mechanism of emotion", *Archives of Neurological Psychiatry* 38: 725–743.

Pelczarska, A. (1997): *Teaching English as a foreign language to the blind: a systematic description*. Warszawa.

Penfield, W. (1975): *The mystery of the mind: A critical study of consciousness and the human brain*. Princeton University Press.

Pervin, L. A. (1993): "Handbook of emotions: Affect and personality", in: Lewis M. – J. M. Haviland (ed.), 301–312, New York: The Guilford Press.

Piaget, J. (1947): *The psychology of intelligence*. Armand Collin.

Piechowski, M. M. (1991): "Emotional development and emotional giftedness", in: Colangelo N. – G. Davis (eds.), *Handbook of gifted education*. Needham Heights, MA: Allyn & Bacon.

Pintrich, P. R. – D. H. Schunk (2002): *Motivation in education: theory, research and applications*. Englewood Cliffs, New York: Prentice Hall.

Piskorska, A. – T. P. Krzeszowski – B. Marek (2008): *Uczeń z dysfunkcją wzroku na lekcji angielskiego. Wskazówki metodyczne dla nauczycieli*. Warszawa.

Plutchik, R. (1980): *Emotion: a psychoevolutionary synthesis*. New York: Harper & Row.

Puppel, S. (2001): *A concise guide to psycholinguistics*. Poznań.

Race, P. (2007): *How to get a good degree. Making the most of your time at university*. Open University Press.

Raffini, J. P. (1996): *150 ways to increase intrinsic motivation in the classroom*. Needham Heights: Allyn and Bacon.

Revell, J. (1980): *Teaching techniques for communicative English*. London: Allen and Unwin.

Rezen, S. V. – C. Hausman (1985): *Coping with hearing loss. A guide for adults and their families*. New York: Dembner Books.

Richards, J. C. – T. S. Rogers (2001): *Approaches and methods in language teaching. A description and analysis*. Cambridge University Press.

Rinvolucri, M. (1985): *Grammar games*. Cambridge University Press.

Rodgers, T. S. (2001): *Language teaching methodology*. Washington.

Rokeach, M. (1973): *The nature of human values*. New York: The Free Press.

Rosaldo, M. (1980): *Culture theory. Essays on mind, self, and emotion*. Cambridge University Press.

Rugg, G. – M. Petre (2007): *A guide to research methods*. Open University Press.

Russell, J. A. (1991): "Culture and categorization of emotions", *Psychological Bulletin* 110: 426–450.

Ryle, G. (1948): *The concept of mind*. London: Hutchinson.

Sachs, J. S. (1967): "Recognition memory for syntactic and semantic aspects of connected discourse", *Perception and Psychophysics* 2: 437–442.

Sander, D. – K. R. Scherer (ed.) (2009): *The Oxford companion to emotion and the affective sciences*. Oxford University Press.

Sarason, I. G. (1972): *Personality: An objective approach*. New York: Wiley.

Saretsky, T. (1977): *Active techniques and group therapy*. New York: Jason Aronson.

Schwartz, S. H. (1992): "Universals in the structure and content of values: Theoretical advances and empirical tests in 20 countries", *Advanced in Experimental Social Psychology* 25: 1–65.

Scrivener, J. (2003): *Teaching grammar*. Oxford University Press.

Sękowska, Z. (1981): *Tyflopedagogika*. PWN, Warszawa.

Sękowska, Z. (1983): "Poziom dysfunkcji wzroku a możliwości rewalidacji", *Przegląd Tyflologiczny* 1.

Sękowska, Z. (1984): "Uwarunkowania procesu kształcenia uczniów niewidomych i niedowidzących", *Szkoła Specjalna* 1.

Shiffrin, R. M. – W. Schneider (1977): "Controlled and automatic human information processing: perceptual learning, automatic, attending, and a general theory", *Psychological Review* 84: 90–127.

Shouse, E. (2005): "Feeling, emotion, affect", *M/C Journal* 8, vol. 6.

Siek – Piskozub, T. (2001): *Uczyć się bawiąc. Strategia ludyczna na lekcji języka obcego*. PWN Warszawa.

Sisson, C. P. (2009): *Sztuka świadomego oddychania*. Warszawa.

Siever, R. (1988): *Sand*. New York: W. H. Freeman & Co.

Siminov, P. V. (1970): "Feelings and emotions: the Loyola Symposium: The information theory of emotion", in: Arnold M. B. (eds.), 145–149, New York: Academic Press.

Skinner, B. F. (1974): *About behaviourism*. New York: Vintage Books.

Sonnemans, J. – N. H. Frijda (1994): "The structure of subjective emotional intensity", *Cognition and emotion* 8, vol. 4: 329–350.

Spaventa, L. (1980): *Towards the creative teaching of English*. London: Allen and Unwin.

Spolsky, B. (1989): *Conditions for second language learning*. Oxford University Press.

Spungin, S. (ed.) (2008): *When you have a visually impaired student in your classroom. A guide for teachers.* American Foundation for the Blind Press.

Steinberg, D. (1993): *An introduction to psycholinguistics.* Longman.

Stern, H. H. (1994): *Fundamental concepts of language teaching.* Oxford University Press.

Stevick, E. W. (1976): *Memory, meaning and method.* Rowley, MA: Newburry House.

Stevick, E. W. (1980): *A way and ways.* Rowley, MA: Newburry House.

Stevick, E. W. (1986): *Images and options in the language classroom.* Cambridge University Press.

Stevick, E. W. (1994): *Teaching and learning languages.* Cambridge University Press.

Strongman, K. T. (1993): "Emotion theory and cognitive behaviour therapy", *Behaviour Change* 10: 141–153.

Strongman, K. T. (1996): *The psychology of emotion. Theories of emotion in perspective.* John Wiley & Sons.

Suter, W. – H. C. Lindgren (1995): *Experimentation in psychology. A guided tour.* Masachusetts.

Sweeney, D. (1997): "Introduction", in: *Carey, L., Sandplay with children and families.* Northvale, NJ: Jason Aronson, Inc.

Sweeney, D. – L. Homeyer (1999): *Handbook of group play therapy.* San Francisco: Jossey-Bass, Inc. Publishers. 1995 *The Atlas of Human Anatomy.* PZWL.

Tompkins, S. S. (1962): "Affect, imagery and consciousness", *The Positive Affects*, vol. 1. New York: Springer.

Tompkins, S. S. (1963): "Affect, imagery and consciousness", *The Negative Affects*, vol. 2. New York: Springer.

Trask, R. L. (1995): *Language: the basics.* London: Routledge.

Ur, P. (2002): *A course in language teaching. Practice and theory.* Cambridge University Press.

Vaugham – Rees, M. (2002): *Test your pronunciation.* Penguin English Guides.

Wajnryb, R. (2003): *Grammar dictation.* Oxford University Press.

Wardhaugh, R. (1994): *Investigating language. Central problems in linguistics.* Oxford: Blackwell.

Watson, D. – L. A. Clark – A. Tellegen (1988): "Development and validation of brief measures of positive and negative affect: The PANAS scales", *Journal of Personality and Social Psychology* 54 (6): 1066–1070.

Weiner, B. (1992): *Human motivation: metaphors, theories and research.* Newbury Park, CA: Sage.

Wessels, Ch. (2002): *Drama.* Oxford University Press.

Williams, M. – R. L. Burden (1997): *Psychology for language teachers.* Cambridge University Press.

Wierzbicka, A. (1971): *Kocha, lubi, szanuje. Medytacje semantyczne.* Warszawa.

Wierzbicka, A. (1992): "Defining emotion concepts", *Cognitive Science* 16: 539–581.

Wierzbicka, A. (1999): *Emotions across languages and cultures: Diversity and Universals.* Paris: Cambridge University Press.

Wolberg, L. R. (1967): *The technique of psychotherapy.* New York: Grune & Stratton.

Wright, T. (1987): *Roles of teachers and learners.* Oxford University Press.

Wu, Y. (1994): "Teaching English as a foreign language to blind children. A progress report", *Educator*, January, vol. 7, no. 1.

Wyszyńska, A. (1987): *Psychologia defektologiczna.* Warszawa: PWN.

Yin, R. (2003): *Case study research: design and methods.* Sage Publications, Inc., Thousand Oaks.

Yule, G. (1996): *The study of language.* Cambridge: Cambridge University Press.

Appendices

Appendix A

PANAS Questionnaire (after Watson et al., 1988:1066)

Please rate the extent to which you experienced each particular emotion within a specified time period with reference to a 5-point Likert scale.

1	2	3	4	5
very slightly or not at all	a little	moderately	quite a bit	extremely

________1. Interested	________11. Irritable
________2. Distressed	________12. Alert
________3. Excited	________13. Ashamed
________4. Upset	________14. Inspired
________5. Strong	________15. Nervous
________6. Guilty	________16. Determined
________7. Scared	________17. Attentive
________8. Hostile	________18. Jittery
________9. Enthusiastic	________19. Active
________10. Proud	________20. Afraid

Appendix B

SANDTRAY WORKSHEET

Group__________ **Session**__________ **Date**__________

Title of the tray__________________________(based on Sweeney and Homeyer, 1999)

Student's name	one idea	several ideas	wet	dry	organized	chaotic	open	closed	empty	excessive	rigid	realistic	dynamic	static	peaceful	aggressive	buried	purposeful	nonpurposeful	determined	hesitant	unpeopled	people	verbal	non-verbal	other

Appendix C

PANAS/ L_2 pro forma

Group__________

Student's name___________________________

Evaluations	September	December	January	March	June
PANAS					
L_2					

Appendix D

<u>Placement test</u>

Group .... **Name ....**

Answer the questions. **<u>30 points</u>**

1. □ What's your name?
2. □ How old are you?
3. □ When is your birthday?
4. □ What's your hobby?
5. □ Where are you from?
6. □ What's your nationality?
7. □ Where do you live?
8. □ What's your profession?
9. □ What do you like doing?
10. □ How big is your family?
11. □ What do your parents do?
12. □ How often do you go shopping?
13. □ What do you like buying?
14. □ What clothes do you like wearing?
15. □ Do you have any pets at home?
16. □ What's your favourite season?
17. □ What did you do yesterday?
18. □ What time do you go to bed?
19. □ What's your friend like?
20. □ What would you like to do in the future?
21. □ Where did you spend last summer?
22. □ What food do you like eating?
23. □ What are you doing now?
24. □ Can you swim?
25. □ Do you prefer tea to coffee?
26. □ Have you ever been to London?
27. □ Do you live in a house or in a flat?
28. □ What time do you get up?
29. □ What are you going to do tomorrow?
30. □ What's your favourite day of the week? Why?

Appendix E

Achievement test 1

Group ……………   Name ………………………………

A. Choose the right answer. (5 points)

1. ……… you like Italian food?
   a. Do   b. Does   c. Ared. Is
2. He …… playing the guitar.
   a. are   b. does   c. is   d. has
3. We ………… Scottish.
   a. not   b. not are   c. isn't   d. aren't
4. This is our new teacher …………… name is Mark.
   a. His   b. Her   c. He   d. Its
5. We ……… in Canada last summer.
   a. was   b. were   c. are   d. didn't were

B. Answer the questions. (5 points)

1. What are you doing now?
2. How often do you meet your friends?
3. Where were you last weekend?
4. What are going to do tomorrow?
5. What does your mother like doing?

C. Build the structures using the ping-pong technique. (5 points)

1. Are we speaking English now?
2. Does your friend work in a shop?
3. My parents don't eat meat for dinner.
4. I am flying to London tomorrow.
5. Was she at home yesterday?

D. **Use the grammar water jar technique to define if 5 chosen objects sink or float; name the tenses. (5 points)**

E. **Listen to the sentences and build the sandtray. (5 points)**

1. I live in a big house with a beautiful garden.
2. My house has four rooms and a balcony.
3. Two people are sitting in front of the house.
4. A big cat is sleeping on the stairs.
5. There is a huge fence around the house.

F. **Find the mistakes and tie extra knots within the tactile knots sentences technique; 1 mistake equals 1 extra knot. (5 points)**

1. I were in London next summer.
2. We lives in a village.
3. She don't wear shoes.
4. Are she talking to me?
5. I sitting in front of you.

Appendix F

__Achievement test 2__

Group …………… **Name ………………………………**

A. Choose the right answer. (5 points)

1. ………… this book before?
   a. Do you read? b. Are you going to read? c. Are you reading?
   d. Have you read?
2. It's ten ……nine.
   a. to b. for c. at d. in
3. They didn't …… tickets.
   a. buying b. bought c. to buy d. buy
4. I haven't ……… this book before.
   a. read b. to read c. reading d. readed
5. Today's breakfast is ……… than yesterday's.
   a. more good b. gooder c. better d. more better

B. Answer the questions. (5 points)

1. What would you like to do in the future?
2. Who is the nicest person in your family?
3. What did you do yesterday?
4. Have you ever been in love?
5. Will you buy a present for yourself?

C. Build the structures using the ping-pong technique. (5 points)

1. I didn't go to work 3 days ago.
2. Have you ever been to London?
3. I am the best footballer in our school team.
4. Will you help me?
5. She doesn't do shopping.

D. **Use the grammar water jar technique to define if 5 chosen objects sink or float; name the tenses. (5 points)**

E. **Listen to the sentences and build the sandtray. (5 points)**

1. Last year we spent our holidays at the seaside.
2. The sea was calm.
3. There were a lot of people and birds on the beach.
4. A lot of pebbles were in wet sand.
5. Children built a huge sand castle.

F. **Find the mistakes and tie extra knots within the tactile knots sentences technique; 1 mistake equals 1 extra knot. (5 points)**

1. We isn't dancing and singing now.
2. Have you ever work in a restaurant?
3. Did you went there?
4. We done some shopping in Paris last Saturday.
5. We learnt English since 2002.

Index of names

Polish Studies in English Language and Literature

Edited by Jacek Fisiak

Vol. 1 Barbara Lewandowska-Tomaszczyk (ed.): Cognitive Perspectives on Language. 1999.

Vol. 2 Marek Wilczyński: The Phantom and the Abyss. The Gothic Fiction in America and Aesthetics of the Sublime 1798-1856. 1999.

Vol. 3 Ian Firla (ed.): Robert Graves's Historical Novels. 2000.

Vol. 4 Joanna Przedlacka: Estuary English? A Sociophonetic Study of Teenage Speech in the Home Counties. 2002.

Vol. 5 Wiesław Oleksy (ed.): Language Function, Structure, and Change. Essays in Linguistics in Honor of Tomasz P. Krzeszowski. 2002.

Vol. 6 Janusz Arabski (ed.): Time for Words. Studies in Foreign Language Vocabulary Acquisition. 2002.

Vol. 7 Katarzyna Dziubalska-Kołaczyk: Beats-and-Binding Phonology. 2002.

Vol. 8 Zdzisław Wąsik: Epistemological Perspectives on Linguistic Semiotics. 2003.

Vol. 9 Jacek Witkoś: Movement and Reconstruction: Questions and Principle C Effects in English and Polish. 2003.

Vol. 10 Liliana Sikorska (ed.): Aspects of Suffering. Classical Themes in Literature in English. 2004.

Vol. 11 Anna Duszak / Urszula Okulska (eds.): Speaking from the Margin. Global English from a European Perspective. 2004.

Vol. 12 Grzegorz Kość: Robert Lowell. Uncomfortable Epigone of the Grands Maîtres. 2005.

Vol. 13 Liliana Sikorska (ed.): Ironies of Art/Tragedies of Life. Essays on Irish Literature. 2005.

Vol. 14 Urszula Okulska: Gender and the Formation of Modern Standard English. A Socio-Historical Corpus Study with Early Modern English in Focus. 2006.

Vol. 15 Liliana Sikorska (ed.): A Universe of (Hi)Stories. Essays on J.M. Coetzee. 2006.

Vol. 16 Kacper Bartczak: In Search of Communication and Community. The Poetry of John Ashbery. 2006.

Vol. 17 Anna Duszak / Urszula Okulska (eds.): Bridges and Barriers in Metalinguistic Discourse. 2006.

Vol. 18 Arleta Adamska-Sałaciak: Meaning and the Bilingual Dictionary. The Case of English and Polish. 2006.

Vol. 19 Małgorzata Fabiszak (ed.): Language and Meaning. Cognitive and Functional Perspectives. 2007.

Vol. 20 Sabine Heinz: Celtic Literatures – Discoveries. 2007.

Vol. 21 Iwona Kokorniak: English *at*: An Integrated Semantic Analysis. 2007.

Vol. 22 Christina Laurer: Poor Paul: L Vocalisation and the Process of Syllable-Coda Weakening. 2008.

Vol. 23 Jacek Witkoś / Gisbert Fanselow (eds.): Elements of Slavic and Germanic Grammars: A Comparative View. Papers on Topical Issues in Syntax and Morphosyntax. 2008.

Vol. 24 Przemysław Tajsner: Aspects of the Grammar of Focus. A Minimalist View. 2008.

Vol. 25 Ewa Wełnic / Jacek Fisiak (eds.): Friendly Metaphors. Essays on Linguistics, Literature and Culture in Honour of Aleksander Szwedek. 2008.

Vol. 26 Michał Janowski: Inheritance of Features in Metaphoric Mappings in English. 2009.

Vol. 27 Cognitive Approaches to Language and Linguistic Data. Studies in honor of Barbara Lewandowska-Tomaszczyk. Edited by Wiesław Oleksy and Piotr Stalmaszczyk. 2009.

Vol. 28 Andrzej Kopcewicz: Intertextual Transactions in American and Irish Fictions. Edited by Janusz Semrau. 2009.

Vol. 29 Janusz Semrau (ed.): "Will you tell me *any thing* about yourself?" Co-memorative Essays on Herman Meville's "Bartleby the Scrivener". 2009.

Vol. 30 Minako Nakayasu: The Pragmatics of Modals in Shakespeare. 2009.

Vol. 31 Magdalena Wrembel / Małgorzata Kul / Katarzyna Dziubalska-Kołaczyk (eds.): Achievements and Perspectives in SLA of Speech: New Sounds 2010. Volume I. 2011.

Vol. 32 Magdalena Wrembel / Małgorzata Kul / Katarzyna Dziubalska-Kołaczyk (eds.): Achievements and Perspectives in SLA of Speech: New Sounds 2010. Volume II. 2011.

Vol. 33 Anna Turula: Form-Focused Instruction and the Advanced Language Learner. On the Importance of the Semantics of Grammar. 2011.

Vol. 34 Sylwia Wojciechowska: Conceptual Metonymy and Lexicographic Representation. 2012.

Vol. 35 Hanna Rutkowska: Orthographic Systems in Thirteen Editions of the *Kalender of Shepherdes* (1506-1656). 2013.

Vol. 36 Natalia Budohoska: English in Kenya or Kenyan English? 2014.

Vol. 37 Maria Dakowska: In Search of Processes of Language Use in Foreign Language Didactics. 2015.

Vol. 38 Beata Wyszyńska: Language Therapy Space. Teaching English as a Foreign Language to the Visually Impaired. 2016.

www.peterlang.com

www.ingramcontent.com/pod-product-compliance
Ingram Content Group UK Ltd.
Pitfield, Milton Keynes, MK11 3LW, UK
UKHW041828100926
8556IPUK00002B/68